If you've ever wondered, "How could someone choose a career caring for terribly ill children with cancer?" or "Is cancer treatment really rational?", then this book is a must read.

It is also a call to action for those facing life-challenging illness—in themselves, in those they love, or in those called to the caring professions. Through his introspective lens and knack for sensitive story-telling, Graham-Pole reminds us that seeming conflicts between science and art, objective observation and subjective narration, often melt and mingle as we appreciate their fundamental interdependence. *Journeys with a Thousand Heroes* is a wonderful book for all who have children, work with children, care for children, or used to be children! At the end of a very fulfilling 40-year career in academic medicine and pediatrics, I only wish I had had the chance to read this when I first set out.

Douglas Barrett, MD, *Emeritus Vice President, Health Affairs & Chair, Dept. of Pediatrics, University of Florida*

John is a pioneer of pediatric compassionate care, and has always been a master of narrative medicine. In this memoir, he puts the latter set of skills on display, as he illuminates the journey that made the former possible. I would highly recommend this book to any provider or caregiver.

Terence R. Flotte, MD, *Dean of University of Massachusets School of Medicine; Professor of Medical Education; former Chair of University of Florida Department of Pediatrics*

In this elegantly written memoir, a devastating early loss fuels a passion to save children's lives. Both an intimate personal account and a fascinating look at the origins of pediatric oncology, *Journeys with a Thousand Heroes* is about one physician's education in love and courage, provided by the youngest and most vulnerable of patients. Wondrously inspiring and absolutely unforgettable.

Marcia Trahan, *memoirist and editor*

Dr. Graham-Pole's book does not offer trite and easy answers, but describes in true story after true story the lives of those (including that of the author) who come face to face with the "mortal coil" of childhood cancer. The children in Dr. Graham-Pole's book take center stage - not the drama and technology of a modern hospital, not the diseases, not even the author himself, but each child fully and completely given the essential dignity of telling his or her own story through the author. At times, even the author appears standing back behind the pages to hide his tears, overwhelmed with compassion, awe, respect, wonder at the little lives with cancer fighting their each, unique battle with grace. The triumphs are there too, with modern medicine making cure increasingly possible—but throughout, there is a story to tell and nobody tells it better than John Graham-Pole.

Dr. Francis Christian FRCSEd, FRCSC, *Clinical Professor of Surgery, Director, Surgical Humanities Program, University of Saskatchewan*

Finger-paints, Mr. Potato Head, play-doctor kits, mural-covered walls, giant teddy bears, a red clown nose and mismatched socks…these memories flood back from my being treated for acute myelogenous leukemia as an 18-month-old at Shand's hospital in the mid-80's. Despite my dire diagnosis, by God's grace I remember only my whimsical friend who also happened to be my doctor. I owe him my health 31 years later. Heaven only knows the full measure of the impact John has made on the lives of countless patients facing their darkest moments. His story will inspire countless others in treating the whole patient with art and humor. It should be read by all, because it is one of a life well lived.

Gena Young, *former patient*

The diagnosis of my son's cancer: the most devastating time in my life. That was how I felt in 1991 when I first met John Graham-Pole. Reading his memoir reminded me how this amazing man defines the meaning of care and compassion. Inspired by his mother's tragic death from cancer, he dedicated his career to finding a cure for this disease. He is one of the thousand heroes that he speaks of; it is because of him that against the odds my son is alive and well. His book is full of humor, inspiration, and hope. A must read for all concerned with how physicians interact with patients.

Val Figliuzzi, *parent of former patient*

In 2005 our family experienced one of the darkest times any family can know. Jarrad, our almost 18 year old son was diagnosed with medulloblastoma, a malignant brain tumor on his brain stem with less than 30% chance of survival. We were blessed to be at UF Shands Hospital in Gainesville, Florida with an outstanding medical team. This was where we meet Dr. Graham-Pole. In that very dark place Dr. Graham-Pole helped up find light in laughter. He came bouncing to Jarrad's room with socks that never match, a big smile, delightful British accent and a ready joke. He immediately recognized Jarrad's dry humor and played to that. With humor Dr. Graham-Pole lifted Jarrad's spirits as well as the rest of our family's. In treating Jarrad's cancer his protocol included bringing joy, laughter, music, art all to help us find our way back to hope and life. Dr. Graham-Pole never took Jarrad's condition lightly but also did not allow us to linger in the depressing situation with no hope or joy. In a sky of shining stars Dr. Graham-Pole was our North Star out of darkness. Reading Dr. Graham-Pole's beautifully written memoir was an insightful look at the life that shaped a truly gifted doctor, artist and humanitarian. Once again I was reminded just how fortunate we were to have Dr. Graham-Pole treating our son.

    Colleen Kogos, *parent of former patient*

I will forever be thankful for all that John taught me, from incorporating the arts into my day to day care to compassionate ways to deal with challenging times. There are few colleagues that can impact both care givers and patients and families the way that John has. This memoir tells his beautiful story.

    Helen Welsh, MSN, RN, *Nurse Manager, Adult Oncology, University of Florida*

An eloquent and courageous accounting of a life well lived

    Judy Rollins, PhD, RN, *George Washington University School of Medicine*

In revealing the immense power of listening, empathy, and the expressive arts, this insightful story urges us all to heed the art of medicine in healing and care giving.

    Elizabeth Brennan, M.D., *Family Physician and Arts Medicine Advocate*

In this vividly written memoir, John shows us doctoring as doctoring should be . . . deeply compassionate, respectful and gracefully fueled with love and honesty. It is enthralling from the first pages to the last, and is devastatingly and inspiringly moving at the same time. He has woven a tapestry of humanity with threads of illness, loss, insight, art and humor. And, in a book about the art of caring, he has created a truly beautiful work of art.

    Jill Sonke, *Director, University of Florida Center for Arts in Medicine, Asst. Director, UF Health Arts in Medicine*

Never shying away from both heartbreak and humor, each page is an honest and fascinating look at the life of a doctor's quest to bring not only healing but wholeness to his patients and himself.

    Rev. Peter Andrew Smith, *Author,* <u>All Things are Ready</u> *and* <u>Lectionary Stories for Preaching and Teaching</u>

This memoir helps us understand not only how important are art, holism, and spirituality in medicine, but how their importance came to be recognized and accepted. It has my highest recommendation.

    Anne Camozzi, M.Ed., *educator, silk artist, author of "Galaxies: Serenity Within" and disability advocate and leader*

John's bonding with sick children, parents, and caregivers brings the reader a powerful dose of humor and pathos. Keep tissues handy. At the same time, be ready at any moment to stand up and dance with joy!

    Gail K. Ellison, Ph.D., *Writer in Residence; Adjunct Faculty, College of Medicine & Center for Arts in Medicine, University of Florida*

How sweet it is that a man can compose a memoir of their life that is filled with loving others. And not just loving but caring for sick and dying children and their families for 40 years with glee. I met John when he was a young doctor using play in medicine in a beautiful and accepted way. And with this new book, his letter to his long deceased mom was the clincher. Everything I love about myself came from my Mom. So John, I stand with you: "Yea! Mom! Moms can surely make fine doctors!"

    Patch Adams, M.D., *Founder and Director, Gesundheit Institute*

JOURNEYS WITH A THOUSAND HEROES:
A CHILD ONCOLOGIST'S STORY

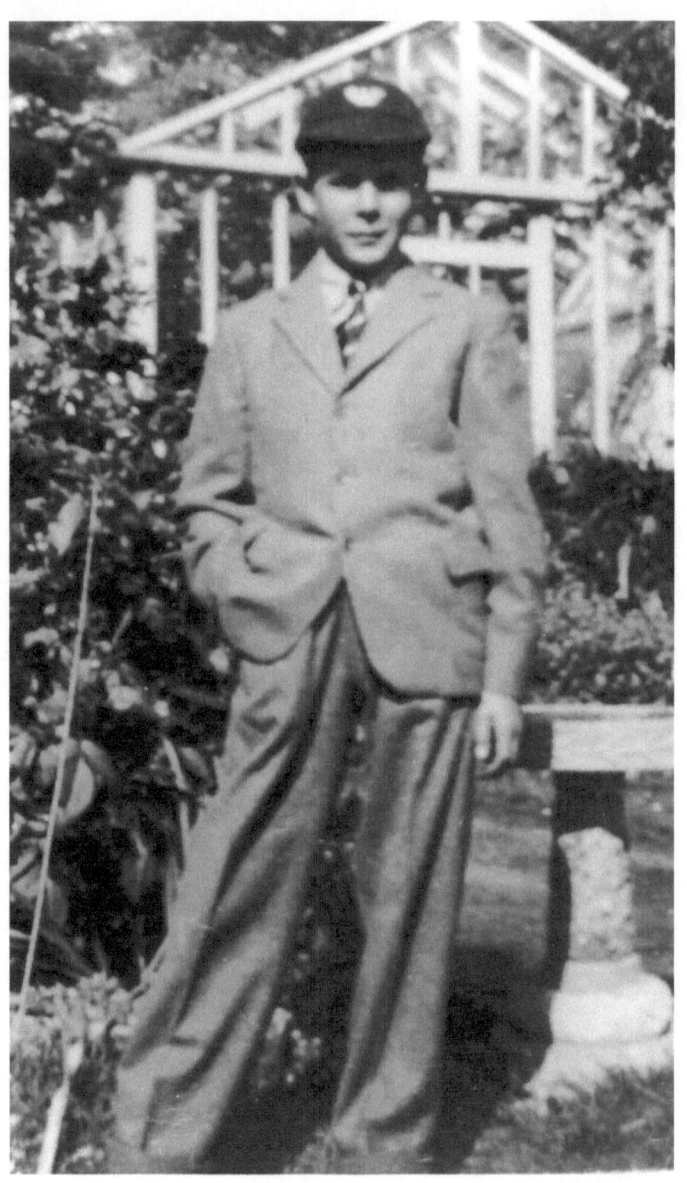

JOURNEYS WITH A THOUSAND HEROES:
A CHILD ONCOLOGIST'S STORY

John Graham-Pole

Wising Up Press Collective
Wising Up Press

Wising Up Press
P.O. Box 2122
Decatur, GA 30031-2122
www.universaltable.org

Copyright © 2018 by John Graham-Pole

All rights reserved. No part of this book may be used or reproduced in any manner whatsoever without written permission, except in the case of brief quotations embodied in critical articles or reviews.

Catalogue-in-Publication data is on file with the Library of Congress.
LCCN: 2018947694

Wising Up ISBN: 978-0-9826933-4-6

CONTENTS

INTRODUCTION	1
Chapter 1: LEAVING	3
Chapter 2: JOURNEYING	27
Chapter 3: MAKING FRIENDS	47
Chapter 4: LEARNING	65
Chapter 5: CLIMBING	97
Chapter 6: VENTURING	125
Chapter 7: GROUNDING	147
Chapter 8: CREATING	177
Chapter 9: HOMECOMING	201
ACKNOWLEDGMENTS	227
DISCUSSION QUESTIONS	229

Sweet as nuts

I began by aligning their bowed bones, learned
the trick from the ER nurse, who lacked the license
but took license anyway, there being no
other mentor. A vain and sloppy art it was:

their pliant ulnas lined up straight whatever I did.
So I learned a further skill: cartooning stiffening casts,
with clumsy craft surmounting puckers and whimpers.

Later we would play as I chased them over and under cribs
for h&p's*: outrageously fit-to-bust, go-for-broke,
sweet-as-nuts playful they were. So where do they go to,
these young ones? And where do grown-ups come from?

medical slang for history-taking and physical examination

Flowers and soldiers

An ill-timed final frost felled my March azalea regiments;
a happening no more rational than the child's death.

Last night they'd paraded, stems erect, my guard of rose and crimson,
shedding their wind-jarred petal-deck to mark my frontier posts.

Like this chosen child they'd shimmered shortly in an early sun.
Now my nursery box brims with their brave residue.

Their soldier paint has run to rust in the crevices of cedar chip,
they who left without notice, unwilling that age should wrinkle them.

A note about names

The stories in this book are true; and I have included the true names of my own family and some of my colleagues. But in other instances, especially concerning patients and other colleagues, I have been careful to disguise identifying details to assure confidentiality.

INTRODUCTION

A line from a letter my mother wrote me when I was twelve, two weeks before she died: *"Johnny-Boy . . . I think you will choose medicine."* Her death inspired my life with children with cancer, who became my mentors and companions on my journey to reclaim—as did Dorothy in *The Wizard of Oz*—my full intelligence, heart, and home. The great irony of my life is that I wasn't to read her prophetic words until after my retirement more than fifty years on.

Witnessing the sacred moment of birth and first breath of a newborn during my medical school obstetrics rotation, holding the still beating cord in my hands, sealed my enduring love for children. This book tells the stories of some of them, and of my own life of care for them. They mostly had cancer or other critical illness, and I tell their tales against the backdrop of transformation in children's oncology over the past four decades. When I graduated from medical school fifty years ago, hardly a child was cured; today, three-quarters may grow to have children of their own.

My mother's death lit the spark in me to follow a life as an oncologist. Children became my allies and mentors, and my writing comes out of the deep well of creativity and motivation my patients awoke in me. Children are artists in life and, faced with life-limiting illness, bring their creative intelligence to bear on frightening and confusing things, as they confront any manner of adversity.

I think of fourteen-year-old Joey, "prancin' and dancin', smokin' and jokin'" (his words) while he was busy dying of bone cancer. He challenged me: *"Lighten up, doc, who said you've got to be so serious?"* and lit my path towards a new joy in my work. Even a certain notoriety for making ward rounds in funny hats and mismatched rainbow socks, sometimes on my bike.

My memoir's title borrows from Joseph Campbell's concept of the hero's journey—one we all must undertake in our lives, however long or short they may be. In highlighting the heroism, resilience, and joyfulness of children—those "thousand heroes"—I'm linking life's deepest meanings, thoughts, intuitions, to our universal concerns with illness and death.

I'm often asked how I could spend my life working with very sick children, many of whom died as I sat with them. Writing this book has given me the chance to explore what about my work fulfilled me so deeply. During forty years of medical practice, children have been my friends and my teachers. Not least in leaving me with the certainty that healing—in whatever form—is accessible to each one of us, no matter what afflictions may beset us.

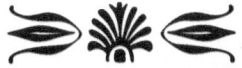

Chapter 1: *LEAVING*

"Don't forget the mint, Johnny-Boy. And don't eat all the peas."

The late August sun slants off the kitchen slates of our house—47 Bristol Road, Weston-super-Mare—as Mummy stoops to lift milk bottles from the back doorstep for the first cup of tea of the morning. Early sparrows have pierced their shiny silver tops for the cream: fine by me—I hate the stuff. An aroma of bacon wafts from the kitchen to my perch on a favored limestone slab by the path to the back gate. I shell the final peapod, brush six peas into the colander, pop two into my mouth (I always keep the biggest pod till last), and pluck a handful of mint sprigs, rub a leaf between my fingers as I head into breakfast.

When I had clambered onto the garage roof first thing this morning with ancient cross-eyed tabby, Flossie, I had seen right across Weston sands and the English channel to South Wales—the home of Mummy's birth. But Weston has been my home ever since we moved from Devonshire ten years ago in 1944, when I was two: an English boy, born of Scottish-Welsh parents.

I finish peeling and slicing the last potato. It slips from my grasp onto the tiles as I go to pop it into the roasting pan to join its fellows, rolling towards Mummy as she slides the joint of lamb into the oven.

"Butterfingers!"

"I think you like me dropping things, gives you a chance to use that word."

"You be sure you give it a good wash, Johnny-boy, or I'll be *butterfingering* you!"

I scamper next door to the dining room to lay the table for Sunday dinner, knowing Mummy will have been careful to lay out the Wedgwood bone china herself. I line up five sets of Sheffield stainless steel from the canteen just so, humming the chorus of "Eternal Father, Strong to Save" from the church service this morning. I relish my new baritone; my voice had finally broken this summer. A lump gathers in my throat, whether from remembering the melody or from the images the words conjure up. Thank God I'm safely out of sight of my sisters.

Sunday dinner done, I rise quickly, knowing I have only one more chore before I'm free to take off for my friend, Michael Trapnell's. The washing up is divided by seniority between the four of us: Elizabeth organizes and stacks the dirties rack, Mary washes, Jane dries, and I put everything away (bar the Wedgwood). I slip half a bar of Cadbury's Bourneville, my Sunday treat, into my trouser pocket as I skip out of the house. Mike and I are catching the two o'clock bus to Brean Down to hunt for fossils and explore its nineteenth-century fort.

No sooner are we off the bus and I've let my terrier mutt, Spike, loose from his leash than he's off on a hundred-mph tear ahead, behind and around us, pausing transiently to scrutinize a rabbit burrow or fox den. We are back at Traps's house just as Mrs. Trapnell lifts her first redolent crusty loaf from the oven. We race to coat each hot-buttered slice with damson jam before it cools, then, stuffed with cream horns and Bakewell tart, embark on a two-hour game of cricket on the back lawn until it's too dark to sight the ball.

Two more weeks of summer idyll before boarding school—Mike's in nearby Taunton, mine in Epsom, Surrey—a million miles between two twelve-year-old bosom buddies.

"Let me give you a hand, John."

Mummy finishes up paying the taxi cab as I heft my battered trunk onto the pavement outside Weston railway station. This is only the second taxi I have ever ridden in; the first was when our whole family went to Knightstone theatre to see *Aladdin* the Christmas before I was seven. Mummy buys our railway tickets—return for her, one-way for me—and we make our way to Platform two to catch the eleven-o'clock *Cornish Riviera Express* for Paddington. A few more precious moments before billowing balloons of steam and screeching brakes announce its arrival. We take involuntary leaps back before I reluctantly let Mummy grasp one leather trunk strap and we hoist it between us into a third-class compartment. It was my father's from his two London colleges, and had come into my possession only last night when Mummy dug it out of longtime storage in the attic. There are several readable address labels still affixed, including from University College's men's hostel and Barts medical school, the latter bearing its black-and-white crest.

My father's name is rarely mentioned. I have only one photo—"Dick and Doreen, Oct 1933"—taken two years before my eldest sister, Elizabeth, was born. They sit close on a hillside in the Scottish Highlands, my father's homeland. He sports a meerschaum pipe, Mummy a picnic hamper: a picture of honeymoon bliss. Did that bliss make it to my conception? Was I the offspring of a moment's union, another reconciliation after more shenanigans? Or was I simply a blip in the downward spiral of a marriage already dead?

He has been gone since I was two, apparently unmissed. Financial support for Mummy is gone too, although he had moved to posh home-counties Guildford after their divorce. Family lore has it he barely escaped losing his medical license for hanky-pankying with his patients. They were said to revere him, and he to exploit their devotion.

The dread day, Friday, September 3, has arrived, and I am on my first trip to London. By day's end, I'll be assigned a dormitory bed in Epsom College, my new boys-only boarding school. Mummy and I are our compartment's sole occupants, so I stand the trunk on end in one corner as she takes a seat on the opposite side, crosses her legs, pulls out Mrs. Gaskell's *Cranford* from her worn brown handbag and opens it at a well-thumbed page. As I hoist my tuck box onto the storage space above us, I take in her Sunday-best royal-blue dress with matching flower-feather fascinator and store the picture in my mind. She glances up smiling, causing me to glance away quickly to hide unlooked-for tears, blink at my italicized surname and initials penned in bold black ink on the trunk.

I welcome the ensuing silence, feeling the chasm opening between us. I am barely holding on, and I couldn't stand her sympathy, worse still small talk about nothing. I retreat to the corridor for a last sight of the poster exalting Weston's seaside charms: *Air Like Wine*—a blond-haired knockout in turquoise bathing suit. I crane my head out the window, letting the breeze sweep the unmanly mist from my eyes back towards my childhood haven.

I gulp down the last of my tomato and marmite sandwich as the guard announces our approach to Paddington. "Don't leave anything behind, John.

You get out first so I can check."

There is no chance for even a glimpse at London's theatres, galleries, and museums as we take the lift down to the tube platform and lug trunk and tuck box between us onto the Bakerloo Line. Jostled in a sea of urbane Londoners, I cling to a ceiling strap and mouth the station names: Edgware Road, Marylebone, Baker Street, Regent's Park, Oxford Circus, Piccadilly Circus, Charing Cross, Embankment. And last, Waterloo—*my Waterloo*.

In a blur of porters and queues for more train tickets, we are quickly aboard the *Southeast Suburban* to Epsom. I am painfully aware of my ill-fitting grey serge suit as I sight countless boys, identically garbed bar cap and tie color, all seeming to recognize each other on sight. My trousers bag at knee and ankle, while my jacket is so tight it constricts my breath. My tuition is to be met by Epsom College's Foundation, endowed for medical families fallen on hard times, so *foundationers* are last in line for uniforms. Yesterday, the postman delivered my suit, plus grey shirts (2), grey socks (2 pairs), cap, tie, belt (1 each: green-and-white house colors), and name tapes (1 pack: *J.R.Graham-Pole*). My vests and underpants come at Mummy's expense, every item marked with its owner's last name and initials. Mummy spent my last night at home sewing tapes on all fifteen items.

We meet my new schoolmasters on the lawn in front of Big School, over the ordeal of cucumber sandwiches and tea in china cups. Mummy corners Mr. Berridge, my new housemaster, while I am left to run the gauntlet of handshaking down nameless teacher ranks. Examination results, father's profession, family circumstances—nothing is off-limits. I fix my eye on my shoes as I stumble forward, pausing to give a furtive rub of each black lace-up shoe against its opposite trouser cuff. All at once, with the briefest peck on my cheek, Mummy is gone. I stare through the black wrought-iron gates as I reach to wipe off lipstick traces. Boys' voices jangle across the quadrangle, distant and alien.

*Propert House,
Epsom College,
September12th, 1954*

Dear Mummy,

I'm writing to tell you how I'm getting on. It's a house rule we've got to write letters every Sunday afternoon, so you'll get lots of them! Thanks for the chocolate digestives and Cadbury's fruit and nut, I really enjoyed them. I shared them with Daglish, the boy you met with his mother the first day, and another friend, Craddock.

I'm in Form M4A. We have Double Latin on Monday mornings, and Greek on Thursdays. We have the same master for both, Mr. Nash. He's okay with me, but he chased Arnold down the stairs because he couldn't conjugate amo amas amat. And Arnold's got crutches because he broke his leg during the summer hols.

We're playing Rugger most afternoons, and I'm trying out for the Under-14's. They have their first school match next Saturday. There's a boxing team, and Daglish and I are going to try out for that, too.

Can you send me more stamps when you send my next tuck parcel?

Love to Elizabeth, Mary, Jane, Spike, and Flossie, John.

P.S. Mr. Berridge's nickname is Connie B, but Daglish won't tell me what it stands for. I'll get it out of him.

Exeat 1: Three weeks into my first term, I am summoned to Connie B's study. I rise from my breakfast of congealed bacon and baked beans, fearful I've broken some obscure house rule and am to receive the ultimate punishment: six of the best. Does he have a favorite willow cane?

"Graham-Pole, you are due an exeat."

Boarders are granted one exeat at mid-term, but Connie B offers no explanation for this unlooked-for holiday. The fly in the ointment is that it isn't Mummy who meets me at Weston station but her younger brother, Uncle Ken, a single-handed G.P. with a practice in far-off Yorkshire's coalmining country. I went there once when I was seven, and was homesick the whole time, even though I got to watch my first television: *Muffin the Mule* and *The Flowerpot Men*. Uncle drives me home in a hush broken only by the gear-grinding of his 1939 Ford Anglia. I relish the silence, having spoken to no one since a brief cheerio to Daglish as we brushed our teeth over adjacent basins in the dorm that morning.

What's he doing here? Where's Mummy?

At home, there is still no sign of her, only Aunty Joan and my three sisters. The mystery deepens: aren't they supposed to be at school, too? After brief hellos, we squeeze into Uncle's car headed for Weston General. My only previous visit there was for tonsils and adenoids when I was six. Coming around from the anesthetic, I had cajoled my nurse to slip me a chocolate ice cream, which I promptly barfed in bloody gobs across the bright yellow blanket.

We are ushered into a single room off the corridor in the Surgical Ward. I hide my bewilderment at seeing Mummy propped in bed in a faded yellow nightie that highlights the pallor of her face. I stand wordless at bed-end awaiting explanation. None is forthcoming. I summon a surly look as Mummy pushes a brown-paper package across the bedspread. I lean forward to catch her whispered words.

"It's your thirteenth birthday gift, John. Do open it."

I rip off the wrapping, gaze at the box lid depicting Field Marshal Montgomery marching his khaki-clad soldiers and army tanks into battle for the German flag, the centerpiece a single bold word, *L'Attaque*. The board game I've been coveting—but why am I getting it two months early? I smile to repress untimely tears as my sisters range themselves on either side of her bed. Mummy murmurs to each in turn, stopping between sentences to catch her breath. Minutes later, I am glancing back for a last sight of her as my uncle ushers us out through the doorway.

The weekend passes in awkward mealtime chat. No mention of Mummy or her illness. The grown-ups find other stuff to talk about without a gesture towards the elephant trumpeting through the dining room.

Exeat 2. Spring term is barely under way before Mr. Berridge issues

another exeat order. My suspicions are on full alert. Mummy's letters and restocking of tuck box with Mars bar, chocolate digestives and peppermint creams, have ceased making their regular-as-clockwork weekly appearance. Christmas holidays had passed with visits back to Western General. One sunny Sunday, Mummy had come home on her own exeat and strolled with my sisters and me in Kimberley Woods. When it was clear she could go no further, we had carried her along woodland paths overhung with oaks, hoisting an arm or a leg each. We had gathered around the drawing room piano, Mummy's frail, silvery soprano leading us in *Loch Lomond* and *The Skye Boat Song*.

Uncle Ken once more stands on Weston railway platform in winter coat and trilby. We exchange not a word on the drive home. There I mingle with other relatives, who offer me awkward smiles. Uncle ushers me into the drawing room and has me sit on the sofa. I stare at the crimson-velvet curtains covering the French windows.

Why are they drawn? Mummy always keeps them open, whatever the season.

Uncle sinks into *her* armchair, that cozy paisley place I had long ago sat astride, listening to *The Tale of Peter Rabbit* or *When We Are Six*, watching Mummy's auburn curls bounce with each twist of the plot. A thousand-mile chasm opens between me and this impostor. He looks down; I follow suit. My heart glimpses something unspeakable.

"Your mother died three days ago."

My heart is deaf. Dead. I wait for more. What more? He is tempered by twenty years of doctoring three thousand colliers, their working lives spent chipping at south Yorkshire's coal face till the dust choked their lungs for good. Unspoken words sink and lie in the space between us, as though he has swallowed grief whole. One image will follow me down the years: fleeing the house, cross-eyed Flossie scampering ahead among the stems of Mummy's undead-headed hollyhocks. I am stripped naked of thought in the January air.

I am back in school in time for Sunday supper. It is so quiet I can hear my heart beat as I stumble between the trestle tables in the dining room. Everyone ducks my eye.

Has the news travelled already?

Died. I've not absorbed the word, not shed a tear, numbness shielding me from feeling. Blubbing isn't in my repertoire since I got thumped on my nostrils in my first boxing bout when I was seven. My first night as an orphan I spend gazing at the dormitory ceiling, floating out of my body into a world without sensation. Next morning, I report for Latin Lit. & Lang. When it comes time to construe Livy's *De Bello Gallico,* I keep my head down and my mouth tight shut.

A mute resolve forms into a fervid declaration of war on that malevolent monster: *Cancer.* I barely know the meaning of the word, picture only a ravening beast gnawing at Mummy's body. I dream of the man who carved her open like the Christmas turkey, jammed his giant fingers inside her, read the entrails—those lethal lumps—and closed her up, pronounced his bleak prognosis. Did he breathe relief at her inoperability, at this saving of half a day's toil? Later, did he stand aloof as he feigned the facts? Or did he sit at her bedside, clasp her hand, murmur the full and awful truth to her, wrapping his words in solace?

I remember the letter Mummy had written my sister, Mary, two months earlier. "I've explained to John that the op. isn't big, and you'll have a brand new Mum afterwards." Did she really have no notion of the truth? A lust to fight burns in me. The boxing coach strives to instill the Marquis of Queensberry rules, but I want only to hit, and be hit. Even friends fall victim to my flailing fists. I relish breaking school rules—turn up late for classes, smoke Players Navy Cut behind the gym, talk loudly after lights-out, stroll on Epsom Downs *sans* school cap. In three glorious terms, I accrue a hundred defiant cane strokes, pain arresting thought, augmenting numbness. An anesthesia that will endure twenty and more years.

Come term-end, I take the tube from Waterloo not to Paddington but to alien Kings Cross. I ride not the *Southwestern* to my beloved Weston but the *Northeastern* to Hemsworth, where I am to spend my holidays at Uncle Ken's home straddling Europe's widest coal seam. I stare through dismal landscapes as the accents grow broader and more alien, hear in my mind the "Devonshire-dumpling" dialect of my southwest homeland. I grow acutely conscious of my BBC intonation, refined by Miss Sybil Athelstane-Cox's elocution: "To the top of the high hill . . . to the top of the high hill . . . my pa's car is a Jaguar . . . my pa's car is a Jaguar . . ."

My mumblings about career aspirations to those masters over tea four months earlier harden into rock-hard resolve. *War on cancer* becomes my talisman, and I declare my intent to Uncle Ken to go to medical school. He does his utmost to deter me, harping on the theme of unremitting toil, and my total lack of any aptitude for science. Hard to counter his position: Greek and Latin are my loves, Physics, Chemistry and Biology closed books I have no urge to open; my bent for Classics rewarded with glowing report cards, contrasting sharply with rock-bottom scores on anything smacking of Science. He rears over me, launched to attack.

"Don't you see? This absolutely rules out medicine as a career. Put it completely out of your mind!"

I glare back, inarticulate. One night, he starts on another tack, rousting me from bed for an early-hours house call. Perhaps he sees this as a more potent deterrent. We hold vigil in a cramped upstairs room of one of the miner's squalid terrace houses climbing like an ancient staircase to the pithead. Each evening, I have heard the downhill tramp, watched men strip naked on their stoops in all weathers, scrub themselves free of the inky grunge with lye soap and buckets of cold water their wives have placed there. How it must have burned their fresh cuts and scrapes, but I never saw a miner flinch.

We pass the silent hours at the bedside of a man of thirty who looks seventy. I tune into stertorous breaths punctuated by black-bloody spittle, hawked onto sheets that by dawn will drape his stone-gray scalp. Uncle pronounces grimly:

"I delivered him. That was night work, too."

Robbed of witnessing Mummy's death and funeral, I have been granted this privileged place at another's transition. The man's breathlessness robs him of speech, but by some instinct I forge brief links with his wife as she serves us tea and a Marmite butty at six in the morning. Two children of my age hold their own sleepy, dry-eyed vigil beside me. I am stumped for words as Uncle greets them by name.

"Norm, Susan, I've brought my nephew, John. He thinks he wants to be a doctor."

They catch my eye as we sit in mute observance together. Are they glad of my presence, or affronted?

This sitting with my peers, as distant in class and life experience as exist on our island, only serves to stoke the flame of my ambition. Midway through my final year at Epsom, Mr. Parker, my housemaster (aka, "Pills," for a habit of rattling odd bits in his pocket), inquires of my future plans.

"I want to go medical school, sir."

"Thought you were a classicist, Graham-Pole. Last I heard, medicine's a science."

"Yes, sir."

I stumble for words, quite certain I will break down in sobs if I try to tell the true story, which would be a totally taboo outcome for an eighteen-year-old Epsomian. But something in my demeanor must have clued him in. He would know all about Mummy's death, of course—housemasters get the scoop on that stuff. A week later he hands me a single-page document.

"This the kind of thing you're looking for, Graham-Pole?"

An announcement of an Arts and Classics scholarship to St Bartholomew's Hospital Medical College in London. Barts—my dad's and my uncle's medical school, and Mary has just finished her nursing training there. *The successful candidates need have completed no science courses beyond O level.* I can hardly speak, finally stutter out my thanks for this too-good-to-be-true gift.

"The scholarship examination is the week before term end. Good luck."

I breeze through the first two exam questions: "What were the positive and negative consequences of Julius Caesar's two invasions of Britain?" "Translate the following extracts from Sophocles' *Oedipus Rex* and Euripides's *Orestes*. Compare and contrast these two playwrights' styles and political opinions." Then finally the only real challenge—a 500-word essay question: "Why do you want to become a doctor?"

If I couldn't find the words in front of Pills, the safety of the examination hall lets me pour my passion onto the page. I tell the tale of Mummy's death and declare my steadfast resolve to find a cure for cancer. I hesitate to mention that three family members trained at Barts, only to hear the echo of our boxing coach in my ears, yelling at me to "Give it all you've got, boy. Hold nothing back." This seems a good moment to pull out the stops.

The day before Christmas a letter arrives in Uncle Ken's mail. He hands it to me expectantly as we sit down to our porridge and boiled eggs. I hesitate a long moment before easing open the seal, at pains not to tear the contents. I read it swiftly, then slowly, then a final time to be certain of the brief words printed down half a page.

Dear Mr. Graham-Pole,

We are pleased to offer you a full scholarship to St Bartholomew's Hospital Medical College. You will enter the 1st M.B. class for the autumn term. Lectures commence on the morning of September 15th at 9 o'clock.

Your tuition and textbooks will all be paid for under the conditions of the scholarship. You will, however, be responsible for your own accommodation.

Congratulations, and we look forward to welcoming you to St Bartholomew's.

I learn later that the funding comes from the exact same source, The Royal Medical Foundation, that paid my entire six years' tuition at Epsom. So my whole education, from aged twelve until twenty-five, will be courtesy of these nameless benefactors. Uncle Ken expresses delight at having another would-be doctor in the family, though I can't help speculating if his about-face is because he will only have to find £10 weekly board and lodging. The rest of the summer holidays I join him on his afternoon home visits.

"Mr. Deacon, I want you to meet my nephew, John. He's off to medical school, following in my footsteps. John, Mr. Deacon has something called hemophilia. He inherited it—like Queen Victoria's descendants. The Royal Disease, they call it."

Uncle tests how much Mr. Deacon can move his arms and legs, which seems barely at all.

"He's had spontaneous hemorrhages all his life, John. You see a lot of his joints are locked in one position, so I can always be sure to find him working on his stamp collection. He'll be glad to show it to you any time, right, Mr. Deacon?"

Mr. Deacon's wheelchair is pulled up close to a dining room table covered with stamps, albums, stamp hinges, and a well-thumbed catalogue of British commemoratives. One glance tells me my meager collection will never be a match for his. But what a price he's had to pay.

"We'll check on Mrs. Kidd next, just three doors down. She'll be eighty-seven next birthday."

Mrs. Kidd is bundled up under several layers against the cold, but she reluctantly agrees to let Uncle sound her lungs. Her granddaughter helps the old lady off with layer-on-layer of garments, eventually uncovering a pair of men's woolen underpants over Mrs. Kidd's enormous bosom. I manage to suppress my laughter as I realize that her head and neck are pulled through the fly.

"Buried three sons, I 'ave, and their wives. The black spit. That's what the coalmines do to a body." She glances down at the underpants: "These were Caleb's, me oldest. All's I 'ave to remember him by."

As we sit sipping tea and dunking ginger biscuits in Mrs. Caulthorpe's kitchen—the last patient on Uncle's list—I reflect on the easy intimacy apparent between Uncle Ken and these families. He must have been present at many of their births, maybe even more of their deaths. Could I do this? Take over his practice in a few years time? But what would happen to my dreams of curing cancer?

Professor Reginald Shooter, the academic dean, conducts us incoming students on the traditional tour of Barts—aka, "The Royal and Ancient St Bartholomew's Hospital." "Arts to Barts for Farts," my longtime schoolmate, George Daglish, had christened my new adventure, in a gesture towards this unique Arts & Classics scholarship that has landed me here. We enter the hospital square from Giltspur Street, just across from the old meat market and the medical school buildings.

"Rahere, an Augustinian monk, St. Paul's Cathedral prebendary, and favored courtier of Henry I, first swung open these West Gates in 1123," the dean announces. "The original buildings were erected over the mass grave of ten thousand victims of the Black Death. I invite you to imagine, gentlemen, the sight of London's dying and diseased crowding London's cesspits, flooding through these ancient gates. Our first mission was more hospice than hospital. These gates survived the Great Fire and the World War II Blitz, and will, I assure you, never close."

He clearly uses the term "gentlemen" generically, given that three of our party are women. We climb single-file up the worn stone steps of the grand staircase leading to the Great Hall. He pauses for us to take in the magnificent paintings stretching up the stone wall beside us, illuminated by a gilt chandelier.

"The artist donated these two magnificent murals, Hogarth's *Jesus at the Poll of Bethesda* and *The Good Samaritan*, to protest the governors' decision to commission Venetian painter, Jacopo Amigoni."

We absorb this in awed silence—clearly the effect intended—as we shuffle into the Great Hall, and my eyes rise to lists of twenty generations of august benefactors, donations recorded in precise pounds, shillings and pence. Professor Shooter adds with a sardonic smile: "Never forget, gentlemen, Barts' proud motto: *'You can always tell a Barts man, but you can't tell him much.'*" The arrogance of the phrase is evident. Virgil's Aeneid comes closer to home for me: *'To learn the powers of medicines and the practice of healing, careless of fame to exercise the quiet art.'*

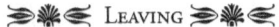

Physics, Chemistry and Biology finally catch up with me. My eyes glaze over the multi-diagram color-chalked on the massive blackboard. Arrows fly to all points of the compass, interlarded with jumbled phrases: ". . . particles and waves . . . field theory . . . electromagnetic . . . superconductors . . ." Will these words ever mean anything?

People are spread along the tiered benches of the lecture hall. Most look my age, but a scattering of self-assured men in their mid-twenties chat idly among themselves in the back row. I pull out the second hand copy of *Fundamentals of Physics* I had uncovered at the university bookshop, along with several others on the "compulsory" list. A hush falls as the professor enters through a door in the front, shuffles papers on the lectern, and taps rhythmically on the edge with the rim of his glasses.

"Good morning, gentlemen—and ladies." He nods to four young women seated together in the second row. He has an Eastern European accent with clearly enunciated English. "My name is Professor Rotblat, and it is my honor to deliver the inaugural lecture of this new university year. I will seek to unravel for you the elegant mysteries of the physical sciences. Let us open our textbooks at chapter one."

Fifty minutes later, a distant bell sounds. The professor abruptly halts his discourse. He has spoken with barely a pause, frequently turning to inscribe more symbols and equations on the chalk board. The only thing illuminating has been his choice of multicolored chalks.

I have felt utterly lost since the moment I stepped off the train two days earlier. Buffeted by the hurly burly of London's crowds, I had finally found my way to where I had rented a room in Tulse Hill from the student accommodation bureau's list. Mrs. Green, the landlady, had started running off the regulations as I clutched my suitcase in the hallway, clearly set on staying a step ahead of any student monkey business.

"No alcohol in your room—we take a dim view of drunkenness in this house. If you have to smoke, please do it outside. Dinner at seven o'clock sharp, and my students are accustomed to help with the dishes. Let me know if you will be missing a meal—I won't have good food going to waste. If you plan to be out for the evening, be in by midnight at latest. The last Number 68 bus stops at the corner of the High Street at eleven-thirty."

Sleep pulls on me as I glaze over rules about turning out lights, keeping my radio volume low, and where to put dirty sheets and pillow cases on Monday mornings. My room consists of a narrow single bed, a chest of drawers, and a table under the window, and I soon learn that the other occupants, Mr. Green and their teenage daughter, Judith, have been tamed by the lady of the house. Breakfasts and dinners are conducted in a silence broken only by subdued requests to pass the pepper or potatoes.

For several weeks, Physics leaves me feeling I have landed in a new gravitational field on an alien planet, where the language is beyond my ken. Chemistry proves marginally less baffling, although the professor's lectures are delivered in one monotonous scribble of formulae on the chalkboard. The only answer is to copy down every last formula and equation and learn them by rote during all-nighters when the exams roll around.

At the Tuesday afternoon lab session, I can barely keep my Bunsen burner lit, let alone weigh out the prescribed milligram amount from the correct jar of powder from the several dozen eying me skeptically from the shelves. Early in the first week I produce a minor explosion and much laughter by adding the wrong ingredient to a compound identified only by its cryptic nomenclature. "Gentlemen—and ladies—potassium chlorate is a common component of fireworks, as has been amply demonstrated by our friend here," is the instructor's sardonic comment.

Biology is almost light relief, even remotely relevant to what I have signed up for, though our first live specimens come with only a single cell to their name. It proves a mind-blowing experience to peer down the microscope at these tiny beings scurrying about in a drop or two of water. I catch myself doodling amoebic and paramecial look-alikes in my notebook, recalling Smudgy Barnard's second grade art classes. The professor devotes a good part of his first lesson to Aristotle, a hero of mine, and the physician-philosopher Galen, who had described the Black Plague twelve-hundred years before it wiped out half of London's population.

Every night after supper I pull my hard chair up to the table to heart-learn into the early hours every atomic weight, equation, formula, and symbol. I close my mind to the come-ons of those bent on honing their taste for Whitbread's bitter and darts contests in the Hand & Shears public bar. At the end-of-year exams, I write several pages in response to the essay questions, but fail the practical completely. "Pithing" a frog and "sacrificing" a dogfish are essential components that are quite beyond me: something about vivisecting these creatures evokes a potent moral veto. But some rarely invoked rule must have extended dispensation to my conscientious (read squeamish) objection to animal sacrifice: they let me through.

Second-year med school casts me afloat on the vast ocean of Biochemistry and Physiology, Anatomy and Pathology, but I'm heartened by their link to my chosen calling. No more rote learning—I've to get a hold of this stuff. I uncover an unlooked-for gift from my Epsom education, renewing my love for those exotic Greek and Latin words that have beguiled me since I first wrapped my tongue around them as a seven-year-old: *Appendicular, cutaneous, enteric, glycolysis, homology, lachrymal, integument, polysaccharide . . .* An endless, delicious feast.

Professor Cave sits at the head of a long table in the Anatomy dissection room, a skull cap derived from an obscure Catholic order gracing his bald head. We array ourselves down either side as his large hands wrap the polished skull in front of him and he begins to demonstrate its subtle articulations. I delight at the unexpected sound of his homely Northern vowels amidst this bastion of BBC accents, realizing how much I've missed them. But I never overcome the formaldehyde stench of human cadavers, remain baffled by how defining every anatomical anomaly of us human beings will ever aid me. How can the radial nerve possibly keep all its seventeen individually named branches busy?

I lift my head from pubescent dreams of curing cancer singlehanded to hone my taste for Samuel Whitbread's Best Bitter, sampling the free brew on Friday afternoon tours of Whitbread's brewery, standing around the corner from the medical school since 1742. Then Mrs. Green decides that daughter Judith and I are growing altogether too friendly, so I take the hint and move into a basement flat in Finchley in North London with classmate Barry Goldhill, the only Jew in our year and the only Jewish friend I've ever had. I relish his mom's gefilte fish and horseradish sauce at his parents' home in Golders Green, a traditional Jewish quarter of London, while overhearing classmates' sniggers at anti-Semitic jokes.

I acquire my first car, a primrose yellow Morris Mini, for £540, which quickly loses its shine, thanks to too much drunken driving after pub nights. Barry secures us a job behind the bar of *The Bishop's Finger*, where we become beneficiaries of the time-honored British tradition of buying the barman free drinks in place of tips. Gangs of beer-deprived students become a blur of befuddled orders and cacophonous laughter, while their girlfriends add confusion by sticking to gin and tonic or Harvey's Bristol Cream.

"Three pints Whitbreads . . . two lagers, lime in one . . . gin and tonic . . . make that two . . . 'nother pint of best . . . three, no, four packs crisps . . ."

Toting up the exact cost of all this gets away fast, but my Epsom College drama-club training comes to my rescue. Deadpan, I toss out random numbers as the order draws to its close, adjusting them instantly as further drinks get appended.

"Seven pounds, three shillings and thruppence, that'll be—make it seven pounds even."

My unblushing authority as I wipe copious splashes of best bitter off the bar with an already beer-sodden cloth is greeted with drunken aplomb. I barely count the wads of pound and ten-shilling notes, plus fistfuls of half-crowns and smaller change, thrust into my hands. All this plus take-home pay, and, often as not, take-home girls more drunk than we.

Then Barry moves us up-market to mix cocktails at the first-night *entr'acte* cast parties at the Royal Opera House, Covent Garden. Kitted out in Sunday-best for the opening night of Benjamin Britten's "Peter Grimes," we master the art of pouring wine without spilling a drop, blending several cocktails simultaneously, and serving half-a-dozen crystal glasses from a tray single-handed. Our reception duties done, I watch the whole second act from my hiding place in the back of *the gods*—the far reaches of the Upper Circle—with Peter Pears in the title role, gazing down on these luminaries with whom we have just had such close-up contact.

Our week's lectures done, I hasten to the queues outside the West End theaters to grab 'remainders.' I invite Isabelle, a French student from Bloomsbury International School, to the opening night of *School for Scandal*, John Geilgud reprising his role as Charles Surface. I relish practicing my schoolboy French, but she proves more entranced at hearing the very best English articulated on the stage. We part ways after taking in the National Theatre, where I switch my erotic fantasies to the twenty-year-old ingénue, Maggie Smith, in *Much Ado about Nothing* and Noel Coward's *Hay Fever*. I get involved in med school productions, acting out every emotion each scene demands, never imagining how this will later guide me in honing my bedside manner. Entering a room to deliver bad news—how fast you move, how close you sit, how quickly you speak, what tone you adopt—is a performance skill that will serve me for a lifetime.

I'm drawn into the annual Christmas holiday shows that take place on the Barts wards, and traditionally caricature our professors. The scripts always become totally impromptu, abetted by the firkin of Whitbread's perched precariously on the hospital gurney that carts our colorful and outrageous props from ward to ward. Most beds tend to be unoccupied, every patient that can make it out the door being home for Christmas. And those remaining surely make neither heads nor tails of our antics, but hordes of fellow students and off-duty nurses make up an untiring and raucous audience.

Barry and I welcome in 1964 perched in the shadow of Lord Nelson's column beneath the fountain in Trafalgar Square, surrounded by a thousand others drunk as we. We've missed our last double-decker back to our flat in The Angel, Islington, but happily several pubs have wangled all-night licenses, and I am helping Barry drown his sorrows at failing to make it through the pre-med final exams. Sadly, he won't be joining me on January 4 to enter the hospital's hallowed West Gates, my head crammed with anatomy-biochemistry-pathology facts and formulae that gust through my brain like washing in a winter windstorm. Barry may not have learned the twenty-six bones and thirty-three articulations in the human foot, the crazy complexity of the Krebs cycle (are there really that many organic acids?), or the arcane links between pituitary, adrenal, and gonadal glands. But he's a survivor, with an eye for the main chance, already planning marriage with his latest girlfriend, Rita, and talking about joining his new father-in-law in his inport-export business.

Meanwhile, I am transformed overnight from fact-cramming cadaver-dissecting pre-med to history-taking patient-touching clinical student, assigned to the wards of the venerable Professor of Medicine, 'Poppa' Scowen, on the top floor of the med-surg block. The senior house officer lists off three patients on the men's ward for my daily care and attention.

"Mr. Hickley has some metabolic disease that's so far baffled even the Prof—you'll be chasing down all kinds of obscure blood results from his research lab. The other two, Walters and Boddy, are both getting over heart attacks. Pretty straightforward."

A cynical pathology instructor comes to mind, commenting on a middle-aged man's heart pickled in a jar of formalin in the med school's Path museum. "See those lily-white scars blocking his coronary arteries? Too much sex on top of too much booze."

My senior continues: "Always get Sister's permission to enter her ward—absolute no-no to simply wander in. Get a full history and physical from every patient, and recheck them each morning before rounds. Check off the results of every lab draw and be ready to present them on Prof's rounds. Nine o'clock sharp every day, including Sunday. Poppa Scowen's a bachelor, so he sees no reason to give you time off—even to get married."

My only departure from ward duties is 24-hour call in the Accident & Emergency Department that falls to my lot every four weeks. One night in late February, I find myself gazing through the heavy plastic Accident & Emergency entrance doors at the snow blanketing Smithfield meat market across Giltspur Street. The market—distribution point for animal carcasses from the length and breadth of Europe—has plied its trade here for a thousand years. It's a twenty-four hour operation, so the pubs stay open all night.

Outside *The Dog and Duck*, a gang of porters has laid down tools from ten-hour stints of tossing half-cow and whole-pig carcasses up onto massive meat hooks, where they swing gently in the breeze. They down pints like the fonts are running dry. I draw the doors apart to usher in an inebriated member of their Guild. He has sliced his cleaver through almost the entire width of his right thumb, which dangles like a dead twig. Is it the brisk wind flapping at my thin white coat that is triggering my shivers? Or simply rank fear? Just what do I recall of the structural arrangements of the human thumb?

We students are urged to stand on our feet unaided, but to this gent's giddy gaze I must smack of an unlicked babe. I struggle for forty minutes to realign this vital organ to his pulped-up palm, knowing my fledgling efforts for a botch. The booze's anesthetic effects persist, although I suspect this scion of Agincourt wouldn't show any pain were he stone-cold sober. The staff nurse, a slim brunette in starched white pinafore over blue Newcastle dress, finally coaxes me into rousing the on-call house surgeon.

Dr. W. is notorious on two counts—scathing commentaries on woebegone med student bunglings, and conquests notched up among the nurse probationers. No doubt he is at this moment deflowering some virgin in the resident quarters. I press the reluctant doctor to sally forth from his cozy love nest to my makeshift operating theatre. He drops a cursory eye upon my handiwork—one exceedingly swollen, misshapen, but partially mobile member—before pronouncing for all of Smithfield Market to hear:

"Whatever you do, don't take up surgery!"

With this scathing *bon mot*, and a lustful eye for staff's willowy form, he saunters back to his Bower of Bliss without having donned a pair of gloves. Astoundingly, the thumb slowly resumes its full shape and function over the next few weeks, crowned with a livid scar from wrist to index finger. Astounding the power of the human body to heal itself, with minimal help from yours truly. There is one other happy outcome: the rumor quickly spreads, verified by direct inspection, that Dr. W.'s companion for the night had ripped his washbasin off the wall. Everyone assumes she had been trying to pee, loath to use the men's stalls down the hall.

After six months of professorial scholarship and seat-of-the-pants emergency medicine, I escape to sunnier climes, assigned for the month of July to my "midder"—midwifery—rotation at the North Middlesex Hospital in Edmonton. The hospital takes all comers, so the midwives welcome me warmly.

"See one, do one, teach one, that's our motto. So we get to put our feet up once we've shown you the ropes."

I watch my first delivery over a seasoned midwife's shoulder. No need for permission to attend my first intimate encounter with naked female beauty, it seems. Thank God my face is hidden behind the mask—at twenty-two I look seventeen. From Mom-to-be's notes, she's a G_5P_5 but I'm too shy to ask for interpretation. The midwife starts talking without turning her head.

"This will be Mrs Stafford's sixth baby, and all her previous five went to term. You'll see in her chart that she's G_5P_5—midder-speak for gravida five, para five—meaning she's been pregnant five times and had healthy babies each time. No miscarriages, right, Polly? My name's Ellen, by the way. What's yours?"

"John."

"Polly, John's a medical student here to learn midder. You're pretty used to that by now, right? Okay if he calls you Polly?"

Polly is too preoccupied to answer, already up in stirrups and starting to push. Liquid runs down the inside of her thighs—amniotic fluid, urine, or honest sweat? I don't know if I've missed her water breaking, but I have the hazy idea this is how the baby announces its imminent appearance. And if this is number six, it shouldn't take long. I'm tense with excitement, about to witness my first birth from a front-row seat. Polly grunts and pushes under Ellen's urging, winging a string of colorful curses her old man's way for knocking her up once more. I wonder briefly where he is—probably in the pub with his mates. No doubt he enjoys the conception more than the delivery end of things.

The baby comes fast, pink and plump, squirming and yowling by the time Ellen suctions her mouth and nose. She passes her to me to lay on the scales by the bed.

"Weight? Apgar score?"

Apgar rings a faint bell. Our OB prof. was my favorite, so I've held onto a few gems.

"Er . . . seven pounds, eight . . . no, ten ounces." She looks over to check my accuracy as I grab my stethoscope. "Er . . . pink-appearing = 2, lusty cry = 2, um . . . good tone = 2." I grasp the tiny, slippery hands and draw her upwards. "Flexes actively = 2 . . ." I listen in the region of the baby's plump left nipple, that of a young woman's. "Er . . . can't count her heart rate, too fast . . ."

Ellen hands me a warm towel and unrolls a miniscule blanket from the radiator.

"Quick, get her wrapped up, don't want her catching her death. And any heart rate over a 100 is a 2 as well. So what you got?"

Baby's eyes are shut tight. I gaze entranced at her tiny pinkness.

"Apgar, John?" Mild irritation, but mostly amusement.

"Er, 10. That's great!"

"Ever held a newborn before?"

"No, my first time."

"Okay, Polly's turn. Let's try the baby's suck."

Ellen lifts the swaddled bundle out of my arms, lays her beside the already slumbering Polly, loosens the gown to expose her breast, and guides the swollen nipple towards the baby's mouth. She roots briefly, latches on, then she too sleeps.

My exhilaration amounts to awe—to be present at the birth and first breath of this perfect human creature. The outcome of one brief act of procreation, and forty weeks of molding each autonomous organ and appendage. A sacred work of art.

The rest of the month passes in a whirl of deliveries at all hours of day and night, with occasional prenatal and postnatal check-ups attended by a third-year resident doc. I even manage to fit in a brief but torrid encounter

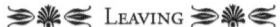 Leaving

with a student midwife. My last week, waking up beside her to the shrill of my beeper, I'm grabbing my clothes when she stirs and the sheet slips completely off her. I feel the strong urge to hop back in bed.

"Maybe I'll ignore that, tell them I never got the call—battery must have been flat."

She giggles. "You'd think you'd be turned off after all those deliveries."

"No way that's going to happen."

"That's good."

She grins again, hauls up the bedclothes, and is fast asleep before I'm out the door.

I've distinguished myself through four medical school years by never setting foot inside Barts Children's Unit. At twenty-six years old, the very notion of sick children sends shivers through me, chilled a few more degrees by Sister Kenton's reputation for putting to flight any student bold enough to tap upon her ancient office door. But such evasive action proves too good to last. In September, 1966, I show up at London University's Examination Halls with the first batch of would-be graduates to discover I'm to conduct my thirty-minute baptismal pediatric exam on a seven-year-old under the direct gaze of my Finals examiner.

My patient is scrunched in a tot-sized wheelchair, face obscured by an outsized mask hooked to an oxygen cylinder. Too breathless to talk, had I the wit for conversation? Two tiny hands the color of blueberries peek out, dark eyes fixed upon me beneath a straight fringe of hair.

"Would you like to know what's wrong with Dorothy?"

Mom, my fairy godmother, has just gifted me my first clue: her offspring's gender. Perhaps she's going to feed me the answers before I've dredged up any questions? Can this be legal?

"*Fallot's Tetralogy*, doctor! Whoops, you're not a doctor yet, though, are you?"

Oh God, one of those arcane diseases I can't begin to spell.

"Um, well, yes—I mean no! Er, perhaps you could tell me something about your daughter?"

"Been sick ever since I 'ad 'er. Always blue—*cyanosis*, they call it. 'Er 'eart didn't grow right inside me, so she couldn't get her oxygen. Three operations, she's 'ad."

Light bulb: keep the lady talking, then maybe skip the physical exam altogether?

"Did they tell you what's wrong exactly, Mom?"

"Never did get it straight. Just this big hole in 'er 'eart. Blood keeps goin' all round 'er body, never into 'er lungs the way it's s'posed to." She drops her voice. "Dunno how she's still breathin', poor pet. An' she has these *spells*, goes all black and passes *right out*. They're talkin' another operation, fix things up the way God meant it. We're awful worried, Dad and me, but we're goin' to give it a try. Reckon she's earned it—not much of a life, otherwise, is it? Well, don't you want to examine Dorothy?"

My meager store of questions exhausted, I spot my invigilator scribbling notes on his clip board as I wash my hands. Already docking marks for some sin of omission? I peek at my physical exam list, fearful I'll forget some critical detail . . . *inspection, palpation, percussion, auscultation*. . . . But Mom knows the routine as to the manner born, responds to my every request without demur. I fumble for Dorothy's thready pulse, which promptly slips from my fingers as I'm locating my watch's second hand. I remember to rub my stethoscope on my pristine white coat to warm it before sounding her heart and lungs. I tune into gushes and murmurs that bear no earthly resemblance to "The Cardiac Exam" in Cecil & Loeb's *Textbook of Medicine*.

Dorothy twists her body back and forth to aid my stumbling efforts, even strives to hold her breath at my request. I clutch at a second clue: at seven, she is three feet high and weighs thirty pounds—statistics even I know are way below par. Then Mom points out her bulging fingers and deeply curved nails.

"*Clubbing*, that's called, dear. 'E'll like it if you notice *that*."

I am Sherlock Holmes and Doctor Watson rolled into one, hot on the track of the baffling whodunit that is Dorothy's heart. I can hardly suppress my glee at reaching a diagnosis, even a sketchy treatment plan. The examiner is beckoning me over. I grin back at Dorothy as I scamper to his side.

"Diagnosis?"

"Fallot's Tetralogy, sir. Postoperative times three."

"Prognosis?"

"Guarded, sir. Chronic cardiac strain. A poor candidate for further surgery."

I've nailed this! But his parting words deflate the air from my tires.

"You evinced conspicuous delight at making your diagnosis. A good teaching case, for sure, but a complex congenital condition with a dire prognosis is hardly cause for rejoicing."

I depart the examination halls thoroughly chastened, knowing he is right. Winded and helpless, this girlie has already faced scarier ordeals than I ever will, and a long healthy life is beyond imagining. I make a vow: should that cherished certificate ever grace my wall, I'll never let medicine's technology blunt my compassion.

Chapter 2: *JOURNEYING*

The words embossed on my parchment certificate, signed November 16, 1966, in an illegible hand by the University of London Academic Registrar, read: "*John Richard Graham-Pole of St. Bartholomew's Hospital Medical College, having passed the prescribed examinations, has this day been admitted by the Senate to the degrees of* "BACHELOR OF MEDICINE *and* BACHELOR OF SURGERY.*"*

A newly branded doctor, let loose on the world. The time-honored motto duns in my ears: "You can always tell a Barts man, but you can't tell him much." It feels as arrogant today as it did when I first heard it issuing from the dean's mouth more than six years before.

I am still obsessed with banishing cancer, driven by the ache of Mummy's memory. I screw up my courage and apply for an internship under Gordon Hamilton-Fairley, Britain's first and only professor of medical oncology. I am astonished to learn a month later that my application has been successful, to be followed by a second six-month internship with Dr. Neville Oswald, one of the old breed of chest specialists. He has built a reputation developing new remedies for TB, which to an earlier generation was a scourge equal to cancer. Lung cancer is the mainstay of his practice nowadays—an added bonus to an aspiring oncologist. The only snag is that my post doesn't start till next July, so I will need to do my obligatory six-month surgery internship first. Reluctant to uproot myself from London, I apply for the only position still available—orthopedics—and they hire me sight unseen.

There is only one orthopedic surgeon, eighty-year-old Mr. J.-B., who shows up irregularly to "do the hips." My first day, Mr. S., his chief assistant, tells me the score. "Two cases max on Fridays—and expect him not to show, in which case you and I will do them. Oh, and I'll see to my own operating lists."

Weird, that eighteenth-century tradition surgeons hang onto of being titled "Mr." Apparently they take pride in this distinction from their physician colleagues. My third Friday, the venerable gentleman appears. Mr. S. is all respect towards him, but I detect an ironic undercurrent.

"Good morning, sir. We have reserved two particularly challenging cases for you today. And they will provide excellent instruction for our new intern."

I'm standing directly behind him as he addresses his superior. Neither seems aware of my presence. While the great man disappears to change, Mr. S. takes me aside.

"Stay well back from the operating table. Your main job is to keep his trousers up."

The job of hauling up Mr. J-B.'s sagging green trousers, together with nudging him gently from behind whenever he seems about to nod off over his operating field, keeps me on my toes. By divine grace, I avoid contaminating his operating garb for three Fridays in a row, and we gradually get to know each other. Mr. J.-B. is always courteous, and I'm drawn to his gentle manner, in marked contrast to that of his chief assistant. I reflect on the sad state of affairs that lets such aging patriarchs linger on into dotage—a sacred cow perhaps worthy of a hospital founded in the twelfth century.

Mr. S. calls me early one morning. "I'm admitting a patient for you. Sudden onset low back pain, came on digging his garden. Numb down his right leg—probably referred from his lower lumbar dermatome. Needs a full X-ray screen, blood work, and C.S.F. protein. Phone me when you've got them." He adds as an afterthought: "He's a G.P. in Brighton—and an ex-Barts man."

My heart plummets. I am already intimidated by the upper-middle-class bankers and stockbrokers who find their way here, always a good twenty years older than me and quick to question my every decision. But this is a first: a doubtless worldly doctor with a large private practice, expecting someone with status to care for him. I can well imagine his indignation at being consigned to a wet-behind-the-ears intern. But I have also learned an intern's number one rule: Mr. S. won't be putting in an appearance till everything is done and dusted and he can shoot the good doctor off to the operating theatre to relieve him of his slipped disc, or whatever.

And what on earth is a C.S.F. protein? I pluck up the courage to ask the worldly-wise staff nurse on duty, field a pitying look.

"It means a *lumbar puncture*, doctor. To examine the cerebrospinal fluid, remember? A high spinal fluid protein level could mean a brain tumor, or multiple sclerosis, or . . . you name it."

But I have stopped listening. I have witnessed exactly one lumbar puncture during my four-year student rotations—a thoroughly botched-up job by another intern. Well, see one, do one, teach one—except that my own first attempt is to be at the expense of a seasoned Barts graduate.

I make a dash for the hospital library, scribble notes and diagrams from a textbook—*Commoner Nervous Diseases*—that has been gathering dust in a shadowy stack, bolt back to hunt up the necessary paraphernalia. I gaze at the alien array of needles in their sterile packages, finally choose three of different lengths to accommodate a medley of back shapes and thicknesses. I breathe deep to calm my nerves as I assemble my armamentarium, only to be interrupted by a probationer nurse announcing that my patient awaits me in the V.I.P. room. I shove my scribblings into my bulging white coat pocket and go forth to meet my fate.

Dr. M. proves a surprise, welcoming me cheerfully despite his conspicuous pain. Reaching for a seen-it-all professional air, I greet him and his wife, who is perched at his bedside attired in a full-length fur coat. Before I can get started on my history and physical, Dr. M. quizzes me about what's new since he left the old place.

Is he distracting himself, or does he really want to know?

"Well, I wonder what year you graduated?"

"'54. Did a couple of house jobs here before deciding general practice was my thing. Lucked out coming upon this spot in Brighton—seaside town with frequent fast trains to London. Best of all possible worlds."

I am breathing easier, even think to pull up a chair—normally a no-no. Over twenty minutes at any given bedside and you are in for an all-day game of catch-up, with barely time to pinpoint the presenting complaint, establish how many Woodbines the patient smokes daily, perform a swift exam, draw blood, and hustle on to the next. Yet here I am, regaling my senior colleague with my own career aspirations, how orthopedic surgery isn't my thing, and how my real ambition is oncology. The staff nurse's words abruptly echo in my ears: "A high protein level could signify a brain tumor."

My nerves resume their jangling. So much for my professional bedside manner. Even carrying out my exam proves a challenge, given Dr. M.'s near-immobility. I succeed in drawing blood on my second shot, and he makes a generous joke about his veins being lousy, though they jut out like tree branches. I call down to X-ray, making a big play of the V.I.P. thing.

"Now I just have to do your lumbar puncture," I tell Dr. M.

"Why the L.P., I wonder?"

"Er . . . my senior registrar felt it advisable. To exclude . . ." (Oh god, don't start listing off those dire diseases in the textbook.) "well, any systemic conditions," I tail off lamely. He doesn't press me further, praise be, nor quiz me on how many I've done. His wife slips out of the cubicle as I pull my trolley up close, maneuver Dr. M. onto his side, and tuck his legs up and his chin toward his chest. He grunts with pain, sweat glistening on his back. I become aware of trickles down my own neck. Who is dreading this most, I wonder?

"Not sure how long I can hold this position. Pain's shooting into my foot."

"I'll be fast as I can. Sorry it's hurting."

I offer up a mute prayer for guidance as I probe for the gaps between his vertebrae, count down to what I estimate is the space between the third and fourth lumbar, which the neurology book said to shoot for. I visualize the diagrams, resisting the pull to consult my notes. I draw on rubber gloves, bathe my target liberally in iodine, and inject three milliliters of lidocaine into my chosen spot. My surgical field at once swells around the anesthetic, obscuring every possible anatomical landmark. Dr. M. rocks from side to side, muttering apologies. I mutter mine back.

"Let me know when you're putting the needle in, and I'll hold as still as I can."

"Right oh. Here we go."

I push my chosen needle in a cautious inch, then another. My patient squirms, apologizes. I apologize, push a little deeper. And come up hard against what has to be bone. A dribble of blood tracks down my cannula onto the sheet as I pull my trocar back out. Bloody useless, the protein level will be sky high—meaning the square root of sweet F.A. The staff nurse chooses this moment to poke her head around the door. Perhaps she has noticed the length of time elapsing since I had disappeared with my cart. Or has she tuned into the muttered moans emanating from the V.I.P. cubicle?

"How's it going in here?"

I grimace at her, grateful my patient can't see my face.

"Just a suggestion, but you might want to beep Lena Jarrett. If you need another pair of hands, that is. Neurosurgery senior house officer. Absolutely the best at L.P.'s."

She glides around to the other side of the bed to assess the full extent of Dr. M.'s distress.

"Why don't you straighten out your legs for a bit, doctor? I'm sure you could use a break. And perhaps a couple of pills for your pain?"

I straighten up my own back, cramped in one position for fifteen-plus minutes, and take silent stock of my situation. Here I am, a newly paid-up member of my profession, faced with failure at my very first spinal tap. I conjure up an image of Lena J. Hot on its heels comes the appalling realization I've been in love from afar with this earthbound goddess since first sighting her in the hospital square. Just hearing the clickety-clack of those impossibly high heels advancing down the corridor, that elegant, creaseless white coat clinging to her form as she passes within a few yards of me. Magnificent—and utterly out of reach. So now I am to phone this object of my dreams and cajole her into executing this menial task, all in the presence of a daunting staff nurse manifestly scornful of my callow incompetence. My self-worth buries itself in my socks. Romantic this is not.

I retrieve Dr. J's beeper number, torn between the abject hope she won't answer and equally piteous heebie-jeebies about what to resort to next if she cannot make it. I cut short the very first peal. "Dr. Jarrett. Neurosurgery. Who is this?"

Oh God, that clipped upper-class voice. How will I ever make it though her actual physical presence?

"Er, it's the orthopedics intern. I, um, I have a patient here I wonder if you could help me with."

"What's up?"

"The thing is, I've just admitted this doctor. Acute back pain. He needs an L.P."

"Indication?"

"Well . . ." The indication is my senior registrar told me to get it—to exclude who knows what.

"Dr. S. asked for it. He didn't . . ."

"Oh him," she interrupts. "He always wants one. They're always slipped discs. You won't be the first intern I've bailed out. Be with you after rounds."

The line goes dead before I can mutter my thanks. I go to break the glad tidings to Dr. M., only to find he's dozed off. Why didn't I think to offer him pain meds? I wheel my trolley back to the equipment room to set out a spotless fresh tray. As I'm dumping the evidence of my recent failure and selecting a new set of instruments, Staff throws open the door.

"Quick, they're here. Is the tray ready?"

They? Has she brought her own intern to do the job? As I whisk my cart back to the V.I.P. room, I catch sight of the entire neurosurgery entourage filing through the ward door. At its head is the visionary Lena J., a model on the runway. Jet-black hair caught up in a chignon, bold make-up highlighting dark eyes, open white coat revealing a black dress cut above the knee, three-inch heels to match. And immediately behind her strolls the unmistakable figure of the Head of Neurosurgery.

Dr. J. beckons me over. "You the intern who phoned? The professor will be doing it—seemed like a case for V.I.P. treatment. 7.5 gloves."

"Thanks," I stammer. "Sorry to've bothered you. I'll just let my patient know you're here."

I scamper back to find both the ward's staff nurses helping Dr. M. back into position. With a silent gesture, Dr. J. stops them in their tracks and introduces herself to Dr. M. "And this is my professor, our Head of Neurosurgery."

The great man proffers his hand. Nobody's paying the least attention to me. "Sorry about all this," he addresses my patient. "Won't take a moment. Just swing your legs over the bedside. Nurse, be so good as to slip off the good doctor's pajama jacket?"

Dr. J. wheels my cart to the other side of the bed, eases Dr. M.'s back forward at a slight angle from the vertical. God, don't let there be anything vital missing. And I'm sure that textbook never mentioned you could do L.P.'s sitting up! Staff positions sterile towels to leave only a tiny central space, mercifully concealing the carnage of my prior efforts. Dr. J. uncovers sterile gloves from their packaging as the professor takes up position behind Dr. M.'s back. In one fluid motion, he pulls on his gloves, lifts the longest L.P. needle from the tray, and inserts it three inches straight and true into Dr. M.'s back. As he withdraws the trocar, crystal-clear spinal fluid flows forth along the cannula into the test tube that Dr. J. is holding rock-steady below.

"I trust you will soon be back in practice, doctor."

I stand mesmerized, become suddenly aware of Dr. J.'s silent directive to take over. I grab a second tube, capture a few more mills of the precious liquid, and draw the needle back out. I can hardly distinguish the puncture hole left by the great man. The whole neurosurgery team has vanished as suddenly as it arrived, the only trace of its presence a pair of abandoned 7.5 surgical gloves and a vestige of exotic perfume hanging on the air.

The first day of my long-anticipated Medicine internship, I make my way up the worn stone circular staircase to the third floor of the Med-Surg block to my home-from-home for the next year: Dalziel ward for gentlemen, and Annie Zunz for ladies. A heady mix of excitement and trepidation grips me: the moment anticipated ever since Uncle Ken broke the news of Mummy's death. Thirty beds line the walls, Nightingale-fashion, flimsy curtains acting as partitions when emergencies or deaths strike. My senior intern, Alan Bailey, and I are in charge of keeping every bed full, bar four assigned to Psychiatry and those that Radiotherapy occupies on an ad-hoc basis. Alan's seen-it-all urbanity makes me all too aware of my own diffidence.

I have researched as much as I can about Gordon Hamilton Fairley, Britain's first professor of the quickly evolving discipline of medical oncology. A rising star of cancer research, he is the protégé of pioneer cancer specialist, Sir Ronald Bodley Scott. Sir Ronald is also physician to the Queen's household, famous for sometimes arriving in the hospital square in top hat and tails—a sure sign that his chauffeured Rolls has driven straight from Buckingham Palace.

Gordon is an eager beaver of a man in his mid-thirties, who has spent much of his career in the States, Europe and Australia, and is brim full of innovative therapies, especially chemotherapy and immunotherapy. Almost all his experimental cocktails are for patients with various leukemias, and their close cousins, lymphomas. He directs research at the Royal Marsden, too, Britain's only dedicated cancer hospital. Rounds are conducted at high speed, peopled with research fellows gathering patient data for purposes to which I am never privy.

Six months on, I will graduate to senior intern, answerable directly to Neville Oswald. He stands about six foot four and carries not an ounce of fat. He appears once a week for student teaching rounds, the rest of his time occupied with his private practice of fee-paying non-NHS patients. Alan Bailey tells me he is a leading member of the old boys club of London's Harley Street specialists.

Alan always stacks the first four beds in Dalziel with "interesting cases" before rounds, which are attended by us two, Sister Dalziel, staff nurses, senior and junior registrar, Ellie, the physiotherapist, and a bevy of med students. Neville briefly examines this chosen quartet of patients before placing one well-polished shoe on the horizontal bar at the bottom of the first bed. He then regales us with stories drawn from his career as a colonel in the W.W.II Royal Army Medical Corps. The occasional patient seems to follow things, even catching onto Neville's urbane witticisms. One memorable gentleman intrudes on these proceedings with a series of noisy farts. "Better out than in," Dr Oswald offers, not missing a beat, as he launches into the miseries of trench foot, the pathology of altitude sickness, and the history of mushroom poisoning.

He always comes armed with a folder of chest X-rays—the gleanings of his travels across the globe. After his weekly homilies, he heads for the top of the ward, draws forth a single chest X-ray, and places it on the illuminated screen. He works all the way up the ranks from students to senior registrar, almost all guaranteed to miss the obscure lesion displayed—though perhaps the more senior staff are just going along with the game. "Tell them, Ellie," Neville finally invites our physio.

Ellie, who has been standing silent at the back, edges herself forward on cue. "I see a small pneumothorax, sir, above the right upper lobe. No more than two centimeters. Although it could be a bulla. Oh, and I think there's an azygos fissure."

"Course of action?"

"None, sir, except careful follow-up. Both lesions are benign."

Neville returns the X-ray triumphantly to its folder, strides from the ward, greets Sister Annie Zunz briefly with "Everything in order, Sister?," and sweeps into Sister Dalziel's sitting room for tea and digestive biscuits—plus, in the case of the medical staff, Burmese cheroots.

But keeping Gordon's medical oncology beds full is my primary task. Their diseases may respond to the production line of new chemotherapy drugs spilling forth from primarily American research laboratories. But they are still highly experimental, and even from my perch at the bottom of the totem pole I quickly realize curing anyone is rarely the goal. Every patient receives repeated chemo courses until the almost inevitable recurrence of their cancer, when they are consigned to "second-line" drugs, of less proven worth and mostly worse side effects. The almost inevitable outcome is their demise after a few months.

With every patient I bury, I relive Mummy's death. From my position on the frontlines, I direct increasingly desperate attempts to haul these luckless people back from their freefall to death, which is mostly from infection or hemorrhage. I get occasional help from Alan or our registrar, but it is unheard of to summon our bosses to our aid—even if we had their phone numbers. I spend my waking hours starting, and restarting, I.V.'s for these ever more toxic drug regimens.

An extraordinary charade is played out in these encounters, as my patients struggle to hide their terror behind stiff upper lips. I get the strong sense that most are all too aware of their diagnosis, perhaps even their ultimate prognosis. But neither C-word nor D-word is ever spoken, everyone seemingly conditioned to believe that their very utterance would foretell a rapid doom. This unwritten code gives rise to furtive corridor conversations between our almoner, our social worker, and the patients' spouses during near-death moments. I am never privy to these exchanges, only to hastily hidden tears during visiting hours. But despite this conspiracy of silence, it is common knowledge that the more cynical among our clientele take bets on who will be the next to miss their follow-up appointment, never to be sighted again except in the obituary columns.

I also have responsibility for patients with advanced cancers that a consultant radiotherapist admits for treatment as inpatients. Mrs. Lane is one of these, a middle-aged woman in so much pain it is hard for her to sit up in bed. When I go to admit her, her jaw is clenched and her eyes screwed up, and her struggles to lift her weight off her back and hips draw forth a sheen of sweat. Earlier, I had peered in dismay over the registrar's shoulder at Mrs. Lane's dorsal and lumbar spine on the X-ray screen: both hips and spine are riddled with cancerous clusters.

"Be sure you have your full work-up ready for Prof.'s rounds," he enjoins me as he sticks the films back in their bulging folder. "And she's slated for radiation in the morning, so make sure this lot is on her cart when they call for her."

"Mrs. Lane, I believe? I'm the junior doctor in charge of your case. I've a few questions for you, and I'll need to do an examination."

"Yes, doctor." She summons a fleeting smile.

"What have they brought you in hospital for, I wonder?"

"Got this backache, doctor." Flinching and shifting her buttocks. "Gettin' worse. Can't 'ardly stand it."

"Can you say how long it's been bothering you?"

"Since Christmas, anyways. But it's real bad just now."

Stark dread stares out at me—she has to have figured things out, but one other thing I know: Pussy foot at all costs around the precise reason for her presence here. Posing direct questions is barred, the C-word totally off-limits. The universal view in 1960s Britain is that if you tell a patient outright she has cancer, you'll be buying her a one-way ticket on the non-stop express—destination death.

"Er, so do you have pains anywhere else?"

"In me 'ips too, doctor. But it's much worse in me back."

"You've had an operation, I believe?"

"Oh yes, last year. On me . . ." She places her left hand over her right breast. Or where it once was.

"I see." I know better than to name names.

A brisk tap-tap behind me. Sister has dispatched the promised probationer in double-quick time: has she already marked me out as a libertine to be kept under vigilant observation? So now I will have to launch headlong into my physical, with scarcely a word passed between Mrs. Lane and me. If I had hoped for much needed practice with my history-taking, forget it. And my exam promises to be severely limited: the effort of concentrating long enough on my pitifully few questions has already exhausted my patient.

The nurse draws the drapes swiftly around to conceal the three of us from the outside world, and helps my patient with the faded blue-flannel straps of her nightie, dropping it to her waist. Mrs. Lane writhes apologetically with my every prod and poke, meanwhile making valiant attempts to hold still. She utters not a sound, breath held tight against the pain. I tune into the bits of her chest and back I can reach without having to roll her over. Her skin is thin and blotchy, and that tell-tale hardness over her left clavicle has to be a cancerous lymph node. I probe tentatively across the jagged purple scar covering six inches of her right chest, and make to remove the bandage covering her left breast. It's stuck fast.

"D'you have something going on under here, too, Mrs. Lane?" I sense the very word *breast* discomforts her, whether from shyness or more ominous associations.

"Yes, well, I've 'ad this stuff comin' out. And it's got all red. Real sore, it is."

"I do need to take a look. I'll try not to hurt you."

I excuse myself to gather a tray of swabs, iodine, fresh bandages, and sticky tape from the supply room. As I round the curtain, the nurse is sitting close and Mrs. Lane is wiping away tears. I bite my lower lip as tears prick behind my own eyelids. I pull up the other small chair by the bed, although I have never seen interns sit with their patients.

What am I meant to do here? How can I comfort her? There is nothing I am sanctioned to say. Mrs. Lane glances at me; I hold her look. Maybe I need not say too much: we both understand all too well.

I ease the bandage off her remaining breast, take in the irregular purple swelling, the pungent yellow ooze from the nipple. It feels warm but not hot nor acutely tender. Infection this is not; there's only one diagnosis. As the nurse helps me redress the site, I am guiltily aware of how much I am enjoying her proximity, the intimacy of the task we are engaged in. Resolutely avoiding eye contact, I quiz her about how often they change the dressing.

"Every shift. More sometimes."

Our first interchange. I sneak a peek at the badge resting on her upper chest, resist letting my gaze drop any lower.

"Mary McKinnon." Irish, but anglicized, by her voice. Private-school educated? I hastily avert my eyes back to the task in hand, slip an arm behind Mrs. Lane's back. Her rumpled nightie catches on the abnormal curvature of her spine. As soon as my hands make contact, she lets free a yelp of pain.

"Sorry, doctor. That's the real sore bit there."

Why does she feel the need to apologize?

"Oh dear, I'm so sorry I'm hurting you. I'll be gentle as I can."

Laying cautious fingers on each of her vertebrae induces the same reaction, more so when I press her to raise her hips. I move on to her abdomen, taking in its unnatural fullness. Not all fat, for sure; her arms and legs are like sticks. I place a hesitant hand below her right ribs; my fingers at once abut on a hard irregularity.

Has to be her liver. Is there no part of this poor woman this malignant monster hasn't ravaged?

"Does it hurt here?"

"It's sore, like, doctor. But not like me back."

Again, the flash of fear in her eyes, quickly vanished. I have heard, seen, felt, all I need. I lean back as the probationer helps Mrs. Lane adjust her nightie and bed clothes.

"Will you be needing me anymore?"

"No. No, thank you."

She is gone as fast as she had appeared, leaving me acutely aware of her youthful womanliness, in such contrast to the other's wasted body. Is she allowed to wear that perfume on duty? Or is it just soap—that redolence of Mom's laundry? I pull myself abruptly back to the business at hand.

"Mrs. Lane, the other doctors will be seeing you soon, to get your treatment started. I'm going to write up your orders, make sure you get something for your pain, and to help you sleep."

I sit in the intern's windowless office at the end of the ward writing up her admission. None of my patients with leukemia and lymphoma are in this sort of pain. I've seen morphine ordered in Accident & Emergency after heart attacks, but mostly a single dose until the pain and anxiety abate. I have certainly never prescribed the Brompton cocktail, that time-honored mix of heroin and cocaine, laced with cherry syrup, said to work miracles with people at the point of death. All I know is that a Doctor Snow patented it in the nineteenth century, and it gets its name from the Chest Hospital near the Brompton Oratory, where they dose it out to terminal cases with lung cancer and T.B.

But Mrs. Lane? The radiotherapists have her here to treat her cancer, so they must see her rallying and living on a good bit. Hard to imagine, but who am I to judge? I am not about to risk their wrath by ordering medicines strictly reserved for dying patients. All I have ever heard in med school is how quickly opiates can get a patient addicted, and that they can stop your breathing in a heartbeat. Am I ever going to feel like I know what I'm doing?

The Radiotherapy team appears on rounds after lunch. I scuttle back to Mrs. Lane's bedside toting her weighty chart. The head chap ignores me, makes a brief examination, tells her cheerily they will have her back on her feet in no time. He scans my notes in her chart without comment and leads his troupe out of the ward. An hour later, Mrs. Lane is wheeled off for her first treatment, wincing with every jolt of the gurney. After the third day of this charade, I pull the screens around once more and sit beside her. If anything, she's in even more pain.

"How are the treatments going, Mrs. Lane? Is the pain any better?"

"Can't say it is yet, doctor. Early days, though. Mind, they 'ad to cut it short today, 'cos I couldn't stay still any time at all."

"Your back, mostly?"

"Seems like it's moved more to me 'ips, and down me legs now. And me stomach's 'urtin' more."

She's eaten almost nothing solid since she got here, and trying to get on the bedpan is agonizing. I lay a hand on her arm, cool and almost white, let it rest a few long moments. I am lost for words of comfort. I had always thought laying on of hands was strictly for diagnostic purposes, never a means for offering silent solace. But it feels like the right thing to do.

The staff nurse waylays me again as I am heading back to the intern's office. "Look, have you thought of writing Mrs. Lane up for Brompton's? She's got to get some relief—she's hurting horribly. And the radiation's obviously not helping. I just heard they had to cut another treatment short."

"Well, I wasn't sure I could. I mean, I don't want to interfere with the treatments, make it hard for them to tell if she's responding. And I thought Brompton's was only for terminal patients."

"I think it would be fine, John. Those doctors aren't going to interfere. They never ask about that stuff, just leave it to you interns."

I like the way she used my first name, the first time any staff have done that. I'm reassured by the wisp of grey hair escaping from beneath her cap, and she's got caring eyes. Biting my lip to suppress tears, I glance down quickly at Mrs. Lane's chart.

"Well, okay. Thanks. I've been really worried about her."

"After all, she's in constant pain," she adds. "It'd be nice to give her at least some relief."

I check, then re-check, the precise dosage of this reputedly wonderful cocktail. I am too embarrassed to quiz Staff, though I sense she would be tactful towards my oh-so-fragile ego. But what if I find my patient dead in her bed in the morning? Would they hold me responsible? I finally write for the smallest dose, but at Staff's prompting make it *t.i.d.*—three times a day.

"It'll make all the difference if she gets a regular dose, John, not have to ask for it all the time."

I sleep restlessly and hurry to check in with Mrs. Lane next day on my early-morning rounds. She greets me before I can speak, and she's grinning—something I had never expected to see.

"Doctor, that new medicine you're givin' me. The sweet-tastin' one. I think it's 'elpin'. I got to sleep last night, easy. And I can even move my legs a bit more."

I have already decided not to tell her the true nature of her new medication—the patients rarely ask about their prescriptions. There is as much a conspiracy of silence about their treatments as there is about their diagnoses. The hospital pharmacist never writes the details on the bottles, just makes sure the patients know how much to take, and how often. And if I keep her on it, she may well be hooked before she gets discharged—should that ever come to pass. I dread to think what the implications of that are, but quickly decide I don't care too much.

"I'm so glad to hear that, Mrs. Lane. Now you're not feeling too sleepy, are you? Not dizzy or faint or anything? No trouble with your breathing?"

"Not one bit, doctor. Even had a bit of an appetite for breakfast." She winks at me. "I could make it onto the bedpan, too."

After ten more days of treatment, the radiotherapy senior house officer announces she is ready for discharge.

"We'll be seeing her back in outpatients. She seems to be doing a lot better."

Not just your rads, buddy, that's for sure. That would hardly explain her newfound cheeriness, nor why she's eating two hearty meals a day, even making it to the bathroom at the end of the ward. I write her up for five-hundred mls of Brompton's to take home. When I take her her discharge papers, her husband is sitting by the bed, a battered little suitcase on his lap. They both have grins for me as I shake their hands.

"Now, I want to be absolutely sure you've got the exact dose of this medicine right. It's extremely strong. Make sure you take it regularly three times a day—but no more than that. And be sure to keep it well out of reach of your grandchildren. Bring this bottle with you to outpatients to show your doctors, so they can write you up for another prescription."

"I'll be sure to, doctor." She reaches for her husband's hand. "I've got a whole new lease of life. Thanks to you, I feel real chipper. Ask me ole man 'ere."

"I'm real grateful, doctor," her husband chimes in. "I've got me missus back."

She is hardly using her cane as they walk down the ward together and disappear out the door. I thought I was going to kill her with that stuff, instead it has given her a new lease of life, no matter for how long. And where would I be without a little prompting from the nurses—a whole lot more use than my bosses. As I sit down at my desk to write up Mrs. Lane's discharge notes, I offer up a prayer of thanks to Dr. Snow, and to Florence Nightingale's blessed daughters.

※

Our twenty-four-hour spells on-call in Accident & Emergency rotate between the five medical and surgical floors, and each one also covers one weekend in five. Monday is our day, so every fifth week we are on call for 72 hours straight. The patients come in off the street, so they are not confined to our usual cluster of cancer and chest cases. Alan exudes confidence, especially with the urbane stockbrokers and journalists alighting between eight and nine in the morning from commuter trains at Holborn station. Their heart attacks peak on Monday mornings, no doubt from a combination of weekend overindulgence mixed with stress from getting back to the weekly grind. Astounding that we humans have taught ourselves the exact time of the week to die.

At 9.15 a.m. on the morning of my first on-call stint, the head nurse bustles me into a cubicle. "New patient. Sixty-two-year-old. Got off the train, hailed a cab, and the driver noticed him slumped over in the back seat. Complaining of chest pain. Pretty clammy, weak pulses, blood pressure 90 over 50. Heart attack, looks like." She had greeted me an hour earlier with words that were probably meant kindly, but succeeded in scaring the willies out of me: "You might feel a bit at sea to start with, looking as young as you do. You could pass for eighteen."

The man is stretched out on the examining table in a cubicle, midnight-blue pinstripe jacket and trousers neatly folded, bowler hat perched on top, tightly furled umbrella leaning at an elegant angle against the chair. He folds his copy of the *Financial Times* as I approach. He is sweating visibly, but trying to hide his anxiety behind impatience.

"Are you the doctor in charge here?"

"Er, no, I'm the intern. The doctor in charge will see you once I've done my assessment."

"Well, I hope this won't take long. I'm chairing a board meeting at eleven." He stops abruptly, draws in his breath in a half-grimace, half-pant. His face pales, and there is a tinge of blue at the edge of his mouth. "Has to be something I ate—I get a good deal of indigestion."

"You haven't been feeling breathless at all? Or dizzy, perhaps?"

"Well, I did feel a bit faint when I got off the train. Couldn't catch my breath right off."

I keep my physical exam as brief as I can. He is definitely clammy, his wrist pulse feels weak, and I pick up occasional skips in its rhythm. I grope over his neck and locate his carotid artery. The volume drops every couple of beats, sometimes becoming barely discernible, and his heart sounds seem indistinct. I fumble with the electrocardiogram, pausing to think through where I am going to place each electrode lead.

Three limb leads . . . left arm, right arm, left leg . . . chest leads . . .V1, V2 each side of the sternum . . .V4 at the apex . . .V3 in between . . .V5, V6 lateral to V4 . . . I think I've got it . . .

Mercifully, his eyes have closed, so perhaps he hasn't noticed my dithering. I spill far more goop than needed on his arm and chest hairs to affix the leads tightly. After a good ten minutes fiddling, I finally hit *record*. The machine starts spitting out reams of graph paper bearing the tracings of myriad cardiac impulses. I tear off about a yard of the strip, then stark panic hits.

I haven't the faintest clue how to read this. Which way is up, for Christ's sake?

I breathe deeply, gradually orientate myself to what I'm staring at. P-wave on the left . . . QRS complex the big wave in the middle . . . ST-segment the flat piece after that . . . T-wave right at the end . . . Is that right? Then I see it, clear as day. My heart skips, as though suffering its own assault. That ST segment in V4 is definitely higher above baseline than it should be. V5 and V6 too—unmistakable: myocardial infarct. I turn back to my patient. His eyes are open, pupils widened in a grimace.

"Mr. Spencer, I need to have my senior colleague go over this with me. But I don't think you have simple indigestion. I need you to rest very quietly here, and I'm going to have the nurse bring a cylinder to give you some extra oxygen. How is your pain right now?"

"It comes and goes, doctor." He is openly anxious now, all bluster vanished.

"I'll be able to help with that very shortly, give you something strong. But I do need to be sure what's happening first."

I barely stop myself from tearing out of the room in search of the on-call registrar. I find him looking over the board where a nurse is chalking up new patients. I thrust the E.C.G. strip into his hands. He runs it rapidly through his fingers, looks back at me.

"History?"

I pause, wanting desperately to get it right. "He's a banker, sixty-two. Central chest pain since he got off the train. No previous episodes, but says he has bouts of indigestion. He's been dizzy, but not passed out. Pulse elevated, pressure 90/60 last time I checked. Occasional skipped beats, but his heart rhythm seems otherwise regular. No murmurs. No other major findings."

"What's he got?"

"The history and findings on exam, plus the E.C.G., all point to a coronary."

"Where?"

Oh, God, where? What are the choices? The registrar has been treating me gently, but he is growing impatient.

"Anteroseptal, doctor," he interrupts my ponderings. "Pretty sizeable. Look at these Q-wave changes in I and II and aVL, as well as V4, 5, 6. We need to get him upstairs. You've got him on O_2? What else are you going to prescribe?"

"Er, morphine I.V., a heparin infusion, bed rest until stable. Gradual mobilization. Er . . ."

We are already at bedside and he cuts me short. Mr. Spencer is breathing through an oxygen mask hooked up to a cylinder, and a nurse is rechecking his pulse and blood pressure. The registrar lays a hand on the man's shoulder, shakes his hand as he rouses once more, wastes no time.

"Good morning, Mr. Spencer. I'm Dr. Thompson. My colleague here has gone over things with me. I am sorry to say you've had a heart attack. We need to get an intravenous infusion started, so we can give you morphine for your pain, and heparin—a blood thinner—so you won't suffer any more attacks. You'll need to stay here a couple of weeks at least, until your heart gets good and strong again. We will be glad to phone your wife, and have her come as soon as she can."

Mr. Spencer mutters through the mask, "No doubt in your mind? Can you get hold of my office, let my secretary know? Had a big meeting to run, but I suppose that's out of the question." He winces, stops talking abruptly.

Thompson turns to me. "Let's get things moving."

He is gone before I can thank him. A junior nurse has appeared with a trolley loaded with the necessary paraphernalia. It seems new interns are not left to flounder on their own in emergencies. As she readies the I.V. and places needles on the tray, I fish out my volume of Emergency Medicine from my white coat pocket. I am not about to trust my memory for the right doses of morphine and heparin. Within ten minutes, I have the heparin infusion underway, and Mr. Spencer is slumbering under the effects of the morphine. I call Dalziel to inform Sister, and help the porter roll my new patient onto the gurney for transporting upstairs.

As I watch the two of them heading for the lift, I feel an unaccustomed thrill of pride. I may have just saved a life.

A month into my internship, I admit my first teenager. It is Jeffrey's second admission for third-line chemotherapy for his leukemia, which means our drugs have already failed him twice—though the usual medical parlance is that it is Jeffrey who has "failed" those earlier two protocols: "The patient failed to respond to first-line chemotherapy" is a typical entry in the medical charts. The outcome is only too clear to us, and perhaps even Jeffrey and his family have some notion, though they are not about to let on.

At seventeen, he is the youngest patient I have worked with. No doubt because of his youth, I find myself feeling secure not just with his drug protocols but also with Jeffrey himself. He seems to trust me, maybe seeing me almost a contemporary. He is a Cockney boy—'born within the earshot of Bow Bells'—and he was already working as a Thames-docks stevedore before he got sick. He is tickled pink when I have some time to spare as the day's demands ease, and he likes to take liberties with my B.B.C. accent. His mother and girlfriend take off to smoke or nap, while Jeffrey and I kick around things far removed from cancer.

My professors hadn't let on that doctors can get to know their patients as people, quite apart from their diagnoses and treatment regimens. I come on this unlooked-for bonus while learning new card games and a succession of raunchy jokes.

Jeffrey is needing frequent blood transfusions, and heavy antibiotics for an infection around his anus that threatens to spread into his buttocks. On evening rounds, I find his I.V. has "tissued" again, meaning the fluids and drugs are no longer running into the vein but collecting in the tissues of his husky forearm. I survey the battlefield of scattered scars among the explosion of bruises, knowing I have already worked every fat vein on each arm.

"Where you goin' to try nex', doc?" the Cockney tones greet me.

"We'll find something, I'm sure, Jeffrey."

I wind my tourniquet about his left biceps, searching for a virgin vessel. Three pop up invitingly, but they have already done yeoman service.

"Nah, not 'em, doc—don't las' no time at all."

I move down to his hands, rolling each faint blue line under my fingers, on the prowl for a miniscule portal. The bruises are even more widespread here, obscuring several once fine vessels. With beginning desperation, I repeat my scrutiny on the right, yet to find anything offering halfway promise of lasting the night.

"'Ow 'bout up 'ere, doc? No one's looked up 'ere, as I remember."

He is indicating the fleshy part just below the armpit, a distinctly unusual site to start an I.V. Open to suggestions from any quarter, I crank his arm to outermost rotation, forcing him to twist his head away. I take in the bulge of his neck cords, and the sweat along the line of his scapula, become aware of my own wet palms. But lo and behold, a virgin vein has popped up, coursing down his upper arm, a good four inches above the elbow.

"Lie back, Jeffrey. I think I've got her."

"Make sure, nah, doc."

Silently, I rehearse the drill: I.V. line full; no airlocks; sticky strips handy; needle flat to skin; pause to breathe; drop needle point; enter vein; check blood return; loosen tourniquet (crucial!); extract needle; strap catheter in place.

A further prayer, and I slide in my nineteen-gauge. Voila! The fast back-flow tells me I've hit pay dirt. Bating my breath, I withdraw the needle. Blood spurts out under the pressure of my still inflated tourniquet. I grab to deflate it, delivering a fatal jog to my whole set-up. The hematoma screams its livid tracers of darkening indifference at my ineptitude: I've gone right through the vein and once more into tissue.

"'Ow's it goin', doc?"

His head is twisted away. Did he hear my muttered blasphemy of blame: "God, why this tiny vessel in this gargantuan frame?"

"Sorry, Jeffrey—thought I had it."

I stretch back, eyes wet, become aware of my senior, Alan, at my shoulder.

"Checked his feet?"

"Nope. No, I haven't checked his feet."

"Want me to look?"

Beyond protest, I push my mucky trolley towards him.

"Feet can be good. Ankles too."

He circles Jeffrey's right calf with the tourniquet, taps his ankle several times to bring up the veins.

"Okay, kid, hold tight."

He slips the needle in. Blood flows steadily forth. In one smooth motion, he frees the tourniquet, withdraws his needle, attaches the tubing, and fastens sticky strips to keep it secure. Ninety seconds, the whole thing.

"Should last a few days. Don't go kicking any footballs, okay?"

Before I can mutter my thanks he is gone. Guardian angels don't hang around for applause.

Jeffrey lives on five days with that I.V.; I never have to stick him again. An immense brain hemorrhage brings a rapid end, soon after we have moved him to the quiet end of the ward to give his family some privacy. I watch them from a distance as they sit lost and helpless beside his comatose body. I take refuge in the sluice, where the assorted medical paraphernalia are sterilized, shielding my tears from the staff nurse who appears on some errand. She stops abruptly, lets a short silence open between us before speaking.

"Are you sure you're cut out for this work, John? That's your third death this week—which isn't unusual around here."

"Yeah, I know. It's just he was so young. And what am I supposed to do? Put up a protective shield so it doesn't affect me?"

"Perhaps so. That's what most of the docs seem to do."

I blow my nose, reflecting on her words. Maybe she's right, maybe I'm just not cut out for this stuff.

Chapter 3: *MAKING FRIENDS*

Ten months into my internship on the medical wards Dalziel and Annie Zunz, I am finally finding my way around. Neville is easy enough to work for, as long as I keep his beds full and have those interesting cases for his Thursday teaching sessions. Rarely, I entice him to drop in on Annie Zunz, if I have an unusual chest case or, once, a young woman back from visiting her family in New Delhi with a flare-up of *falciparum* malaria.

She knows exactly what her problem is and simply wants a refill of antimalarials, having no G.P. of her own. Being a Wednesday night, I had prevailed on her to come in for closer observation. I even have her blood slides on Thursday morning for Neville to demonstrate the malarial parasites as he dilates on his years in the tropics. That evening, she threatens to leave *AMA*—"against medical advice." She looks in radiant health, and her husband is making noises down the phone in an accent unintelligible but fierce, so I discharge her with a two-week chloroquine prescription, and the fervent hope she will quickly get herself registered with a G.P..

I no longer have first-line responsibility for Gordon's patients, but Neville's urgent patients mostly have well advanced lung cancer, so I put in frequent requests for thoracic surgery consults. These are usually followed by frequent radiotherapy consults, the surgeons having biopsied the lung lesion and delivered their judgment that it is inoperable. The chemotherapy we give Gordon's patients is impotent against lung cancer, so palliative radiotherapy is all we have to offer these sad old men. Sister Dalziel knows the score all too well, and allows the ones still ambulant to head down to the square to puff their Player's Navy Cut as a kind of palliation.

I come up for air, wondering what to do next. To pursue my medical oncology career, I must compete for a senior house officer position at the Royal Marsden or Hammersmith Hospitals, or the Royal Brompton Chest for an exclusive diet of lung cancer. This to be followed by a fellowship devoted entirely to obscure cancer research in a "rat lab." Then what? A year or more in Boston or New York to get my coveted *BTA—Been to America—*certificate. Even at the end of this arduous trial by fire, I would be competing with a fast-growing horde of hot-shots for a tiny pool of faculty positions throughout the length and breadth of the country. I don't have to be reminded that Gordon is still Britain's only professor of medical oncology.

All of which is beside the point. I am six months into my new marriage to Ruth, a nurse I had met as a final-year med student, and my job is already straining our relationship. I am expending all my energies and emotions dealing with the death toll—lung cancer patients dead of exhaustion from hawking up blood, leukemia patients perishing from uncontrollable infections or relentless bowel hemorrhages. With every death, my absurd resolve to find a cure for cancer is thrown in my face.

I am dog-tired, can process nothing. Burying patients hand-over-fist is worse than futile. Talking to other docs about it seems out of the question. The nurses have some inkling, but all I know about relating to women is sex—as a means to transiently still my loneliness and sense of failure. At home, I find myself eager for comfort food washed down with several pints of Whitbreads, before falling asleep in front of the telly. I know Ruth wants to hear about my day, but I feel perversely unwilling to share my feelings. When we do talk, we end up fighting and going to bed with a foot of mattress between us.

It will be ten more years before I start coming to terms with my emotional state, and how I can set about healing a psyche arrested before I had hit my teens.

Late in the year, I sit with Neville in our accustomed armchairs after chocolate biscuits and strong tea, enjoying a cheroot as a digestive aid.

"Sir, might I seek your counsel? The thing is, I'm not sure I'm cut out for a career in oncology."

"What's on your mind, Graham-Pole?" He is gazing at smoke rings heading towards the lampshade.

"Well, I started out with high hopes. But I think perhaps I was mistaken."

"What does Hamilton-Fairley say?"

"I . . . er . . . I haven't talked to him."

"What d'you have in mind? G.P., I suppose?" I hear the barely disguised scorn in his voice. General practice is at the very bottom of the hierarchy. But my mind lights on that G.P. from Brighton: "Best of all possible worlds—seaside town with frequent fast trains to London." Not such a bad prospect.

"Yes, I think so, sir."

"I see. Well, you'll need pediatrics. I'll have a word with Sister K." Then he adds as an afterthought, "and I'll mention it to the pediatric men, of course."

Sister Kenton, the scourge of a generation of students. I think back to the first child I ever examined in my Finals viva voce, after my steadfast avoidance of the children's ward. Rumor has it a growing number of children with leukemia are finding their way there, which has become a kind of hospice, with no doctor having the temerity to test the new chemo protocols on them. Six months of that? My mind blanches at the thought.

"Sir, I think perhaps I need a broader experience than I would be exposed to there."

The barely disguised scorn turns to dismissal. "Well, I'll leave you to look around. No doubt there are jobs to be found in the home counties." He stubs out his cheroot in the ashtray, rises to his stooping six foot four, and sweeps out of the office without a backward glance, leaving me with decidedly mixed emotions.

Neville, despite his condescension, has hit the mark. Setting out as a G.P., with my sole experience of children the North Middlesex labor & delivery room and my Finals viva voce, is a stretch. But the thought of six months, possibly a year, spent caring exclusively for sick children, many of whom may never grow to adulthood, fills me with dread. Perhaps I can wing it, find a practice where child patients are in the minority, pick up whatever I need to know from senior colleagues? Or learn fast from the mothers, the way I had in Finals?

That night I pore over the Classified section of the *British Medical Journal*, but find an unexpected dearth of pediatric house jobs around London. I am late applying, so they must all have been snapped up. About to turn to the section on available G.P. jobs, a small advertisement catches my eye.

Senior House Officer in General Pediatrics, Jenny Lind Children's Hospital, Norwich. 3 positions available July 1. Delightful rural setting near the Norfolk coast. Single and married accommodation, and all meals included.

My mind flashes on my dad's tales of sailing holidays on the Norfolk

Broads, the unspoiled coastline and nature reserves. Accommodation and meals included? I realize how sick I am of stodgy rushed meals in our squalid flat in Islington and the pomposity of the "Royal and Ancient"—my sole exposure to medicine for the past eight years. I talk to Ruth about my plans, and get the strong inkling that she, too, will be glad of a break from the big city. I post my application to a Dr. John Quinton next morning.

A month later, I say farewell to my two bosses and nursing sisters, point our ten-year-old Hillman Imp up the A.11 towards the Fen Country, and at five-thirty that afternoon am ringing the hospital door bell. The place resembles a Victorian country home, but the plaque on the wall above—"Dedicated to our beloved benefactor, the famed opera singer, Jenny Lind"—confirms we are at the right place. A middle-aged lady in a kitchen apron swings open the door.

"I'm Mrs. Butcher, the cook. Just putting your tea on the table." She bustles Ruth and me into an airy room looking out onto parkland. The dinner table is set for six, but we are the only ones here. "This is the doctor's dining room, but wives are always welcome if you let me know you'll be in. Roast chicken suit you all right? I'll be back directly to take you on your tour."

We dig into chicken, roast potatoes, and assorted veggies, and after large bowls of banana pudding our cook is back with a gentleman, also of middle years. "My old man, does the odd jobs around here, grows the veg, gets under my feet. He'll help you with your luggage, show you your flat." This last directed to Ruth, while her husband disappears as fast as he appeared, grasping our bags from beside the dining room door. "You best follow him, dearie. He doesn't let the grass grow under his feet! I'll look after your husband, don't you worry."

She leads me down a passageway running the length of the building to a hospital ward out of a story book. It is filled with higgledy-piggledy beds of all sizes, far removed from the apple-pie order I am long accustomed to. Half-a-dozen adult-sized ones are fanned out facing the French windows with a view of the garden, two occupied with chatting teenaged girls and one with a third, a boy of about twelve strung up on a hoist, his leg encased in plaster. The ward center is occupied by a circle of cots, and the remaining floor space with a clutter of toys and games. Two nurses are talking at a desk; one has a toddler perched on her knee engrossed in a picture book, while the other pours spoonfuls of pink medicine from a bottle. She hands the first spoon to another youngster at the front of a short queue. There are more scampering children in rompers, who pause occasionally to engage themselves in the treasure trove on the floor. There is no sign of anyone being ready for bed.

I am taking in this cheery scene when a two-year-old detaches himself from the bustle and advances towards me, arms outstretched. The unspoken message couldn't be clearer. How did I get to be twenty-seven and never pick up a child? I drop to a clumsy kneel, sparing a thought for my brand new suit as he clambers into my arms. I become aware of his sticky bib—generously coated with ice cream? rice pudding?—pressed against my tie. I catch myself hugging him right back, relishing a surge of sweet-as-nuts joyfulness.

Mrs. Butcher ruffles his dark curls. "Probably one of your theater cases for tomorrow, doctor."

Theater? As in operating theater? Those long-ago words—"Whatever you do, don't take up surgery"—resound in my ears. Mrs. Butcher senses my surprise.

"Circs—circumcisions, that is," she goes on. "The junior doctors do 'em all. Don't look so worried, my love, the nurses'll show you how."

"I thought they did that at birth."

"Heavens, dearie, they're much choosier nowadays. Only do the ones the doctors think essential."

Mrs. Butcher seems remarkably well informed for a cook, but maybe she's got things wrong. One of the nurses approaches.

"You must be one of the new house officers. Janice Salter, staff nurse on duty tonight. We've got some patients for you to check over." She takes in the horde of scampering children, not a whit resembling my desperately sick patients of the past year. "We'll settle them in their cots so you can do your exams. The mums are all here."

All six children seem totally healthy, and their physicals are a whole lot easier than when conducted under the eagle eye of an invigilator. But Mrs. Butcher's prediction proves dead-on. My hour of trial arrives at eight o'clock next morning. I enter the operating theater changing room to find I'm the only possible surgeon in sight. Blanking on the requisite scrub time, I soap from finger tips to armpits for ten minutes-plus, before pushing backwards into the operating room itself, an initiate at the dance. I sense a certain impatience to strike up the band as I take my place at table and contemplate the sleeping tot beneath the gas man's eye.

I feel hands fumbling at me from behind, and twist my head. Are my trousers falling down? It turns out to be the circulating nurse who is tying my gown at waist and neck. She opens the glove wrapper, and as I grasp and don the contents, I swivel back to the sight of my scrubbed-in partner anointing the tiny penis and environs with Betadine. She encases the whole in sterile green, leaving me a two-inch operating field, then hands me a miniscule scalpel. She finally breaks the silence.

"Probably didn't tell you to expect this. Fear not, I've trained a few housemen in my time."

Nurses instructing doctors? Is this even legal? I look up from eying my patient's willy, sense the smirk beneath the mask, and spot wisps of white hair escaping beneath her cap. I am ready to obey any orders she delivers.

"You're going to slit his foreskin open, doctor. Right here."

I snip tentatively along the back of the tiny pecker.

"Push back with your fingers, so just his little knob sticks out. The business end, you might call it."

There is a vaguely disturbing intimacy about this whole business—the motherly nurse, the little boy's appendage, and me. Am I cutting into this mite's future pleasure? I comply as she plucks a diminutive plastic ring from her arsenal of surgical gadgets.

"Now draw his foreskin over the top of this thingy." She skillfully guides my hesitant hands. "Tie this ligature round to staunch the blood when you chop it off."

I have no idea where I'm going with all this, can only assume she means the foreskin, not the whole organ. Sweat trickles down my forehead as I pull the nylon tight. I flash back to that bloody misshapen thumb in Barts Accident & Emergency: that thumb and this penis are about of a size. She hands me miniscule surgical scissors. I can barely squeeze a finger and thumb tip through the loops.

"Now, the coup de grace! Lop it off!"

The tiny integument plops into her waiting basin. She cocoons the remaining member in bandage, leaving a centimeter sticking out.

"Well done, doctor!"

"Can't claim much credit."

"Nonsense! See one, do one, teach one. You'll be a pro in no time."

Sure enough, the remaining circs get steadily easier, and by morning's end I feel like I could teach the whole thing without guidance. What the moms will think remains to be seen.

I emerge from my triumph in the operating theater in time for lunch with my colleagues. Mrs. Butcher is again in lively attendance, and I half expect her to take her place at top of the table. There are two consultant pediatricians. Dr. Quinton is the senior, six foot and ramrod straight as a soldier, with a shock of white hair and matching moustache. Dr. Jones is a quick-talking, quick-moving Welshman, a neonatology specialist just arrived from Newcastle-upon-Tyne. There is also a registrar, Martin Addy, and two more senior house officers, Stephen and another John, also brand new to Pediatrics. Dr. Quinton—"Quint"—gives us the rundown over roast beef and Yorkshire pudding about the hospital's history, our primary duties, and how to reach the surgeons and anesthetists at the main Norfolk & Norwich hospital near the city's center.

"We'll be setting you short essays each week. We have a library next to the dining room, but you might want to get your own copy of Hutchison's *Pediatrics*. We'll have you primed for the D.C.H. before we are done."

The Diploma of Child Health—an essential ticket for anyone embarking on a pediatric career. I like the idea of boning up on Quint's essay questions—my recent bosses never saw teaching as a priority. He announces a hospital tour, and we meet the Sisters of the medical and surgical wards, who lay down the welcome carpet. Hordes of teens-to-tots once more, mostly treating the place as home-from-home. Entering the medical ward, I almost trip over our self-appointed greeter—a boy in a wheelchair. Anywhere between six and ten, with a barrel-shaped chest, dusky lips, and constant cough, he pauses from his hacking to smirk at me.

"C.F., I've got, doctor. Heard of it, have you?" He takes in my blank look. "Cystic Fibrosis. I'm in for my antibiotics. In there, they are." He points with his free hand at the bottle of I.V. fluid.

"For your chest, is it?"

If my ignorance astonishes him, he has the grace to hide it.

"Mom gives me my physio three times a day, helps get my spit up. But the nurses do it when I'm in here, so she gets a break."

"Seems like you know a lot about cystic fibrosis. More than me, I'll bet."

"Well, I've had it since I was born, so I've picked up a few things," he answers airily. "Dr. Quinton, he makes sure we learn all about it."

"So how old are you?"

"Twelve this month." He adds unnecessarily, "Small for my age. I have to take this enzyme every meal time, helps my digestion, otherwise I get the runs something awful. Real smelly too. I'll teach you all about it."

"That'd be great. I'll bring my notebook next time. So what's your name?"

"Tim. What's yours?"

"John. You can use my first name if you want." I realize the rest of our party has reached the end of the ward. "Sorry, got to go, Tim. I'll come back and chat later."

I won't have much need for a textbook with teachers like Tim. Quint has paused in the bay window, and we form a semi-circle around him. "Jenny Lind was only the second hospital in the country dedicated to caring for children," he announces. "She was a Swedish opera singer who came to Norwich to give concerts, and used the money to found the hospital. 1853, a year after Great Ormond Street. We try to make this a friendly and, as far as possible, happy place. Of course, the children themselves help a lot with that. Are you all planning a career in Pediatrics?"

I'm standing on his immediate right, so he addresses me first. I hesitate.

"Well, sir, until last night, I thought I was heading for general practice. Both my father and uncle were G.P.s. I was thinking about this giving me experience with children, but maybe I'll change my mind."

What am I saying? Spend my life looking after sick children? Am I serious, after less than twenty-four hours? But hearing my words aloud gives them conviction. I think of Goethe: "Whatever you dream, begin it, boldness has power and magic in it."

"Your first essay topic will be on cystic fibrosis," Quint tells us. "Etiology, signs and symptoms, diagnosis, treatment, prognosis. Let me have them on Monday morning."

That night, I research all there is to know about C.F. How it is passed on in the parents' genes, the chloride test for diagnosing it from a baby's sweat, the damage it does to lungs and intestines—and several more organs, if they live long enough. Then I read about its prognosis. Tim will be lucky to make it through his teens, and then only by getting chest physio several times daily, plus courses of I.V. antibiotics at first signs of pneumonia. I wonder if he knows what's in store?

I go back to talk to him after rounds next day. "Tim, I have to write an essay on C.F. Maybe you could help me. You're the first boy I've ever met with it."

"So what d'you want to know?"

"Well, when did they find out about it?"

"I was an itty-bitty baby. My big sister, Mary Anne, she got it, but she died when she was seventeen, so then they tested me. My brother, Des, he's in high school, but he doesn't have it. Finding out about it early on's good, 'cos they started treating me right off."

"How often do you have to come into hospital?"

"Every couple of months. More in winter, more infections then."

"Can you eat anything you like?"

"Pretty much. Long as I take my pancrex."

A coughing attack stops him short. He grabs a box of tissues and hawks up sticky spit. I wait for the paroxysm to pass, framing my next question.

"So how's life at home? And school?"

"Okay. I mean, I've got friends and all, and I know some of the other kids with C.F. Dr. Quinton has a special clinic for us, and our mums talk about stuff together. I know all the nurses and docs, too, and when I'm in here, I get lessons from this teacher."

We talk for a few more minutes, until I see he's tiring. I'm saddened by thinking about what his future holds, but excited to make the link—more like friendship than the strictly professional relationship I'm used to. I decide to include some of his comments in my essay.

But I am not destined to avoid the role of surgeon. We take turns covering Jenny Lind's Accident & Emergency, dealing with cuts and grazes, dislodged joints and bowed bones sustained in playgrounds and backyards or from bicycle wipeouts. Rosemary, the A.&E. nurse, teaches me the art of straightening greenstick fractures, named for the 'greener' nature of children's bones. She proves infinitely tactful towards my easily bruised ego, just as she must have been with a generation of budding pediatricians. Often, all that is needed is a cast, and the bent bone aligns flawlessly into its pristine shape. Applying the plaster of Paris is a marvelously sloppy task. Rosemary dips lengths of cotton bandage into the goop and hands me one end. My job is to wind it just tight enough around the squirming forearm or shin before it sets too hard and is rendered useless. The younger ones send up cacophonies of screams and howls—more from fear than pain—seeing no reason to restrain their feelings. But once it's done they chatter and laugh as if nothing has happened.

I disguise the casts' roughness and puckers with cartoons in unheard-of combinations from Rosemary's store of colored pens. Suddenly I'm an artist. And unlike grown-ups, who judge a surgeon's skill from the fineness of their scar, all these children exact is my signature. Another treaty signed in poster paint. How many years has it been since I had such fun? Once each task is complete, I reward myself with a stroll beyond the A.&E. doors to smoke a Player's Navy Cut, breathing in the air of that salty coast and tuning into the screeches of terns and herring gulls.

I go all out to perform my tasks as adeptly as possible. Drawing blood samples through a baby's 'soft spot'—the anterior fontanelle overlying the sagittal sinus under the skull. Starting I.V.'s on wriggling toddlers by knowing just where the veins lie under pudgy backs of hands. Performing fast in-and-out lumbar punctures in toddlers with the telltale signs of meningitis—raging fever, delirium, and a neck you can't flex for love or money. The secret is to have the nurse keep the squirming patient curled up securely, so their supple lumbar spines spread out and make the task easy.

But how I hate the task of wounding these fragile beings, certain the traumas I inflict they will carry to their grave—as will I. But the rites of passage must be marked if I am to become seasoned as a doctor. I must inflict instant suffering on bodies and psyches to forestall later problems. Yet how much can a preschooler understand when two nurses have to hold her down as I fail to draw blood after a third try? And what about the teenagers? Do they have any right to refuse what we decide is in their best interests?

I think back to all those cancer patients on Dalziel and Annie Zunz. They went along with all those awful treatments that only delayed the inevitable. Did the end—learning a fraction more about our experimental chemotherapy regimens—justify our means? So how much harder for children, who have no legal right to refuse treatment. If ethical issues are tough in the world of adult medicine, how much more so when it comes to young ones.

But my patients' complaints are forthright and short lived. Along with the nurses, the children are becoming my quite unlicensed mentors in teaching me medicine's art. And who better qualified? I find myself falling for every one of these resilient and forgiving young people.

In my third week at Jenny Lind, Martin Addy admits five-year-old Audrey from his clinic with a fever of 102. She lies motionless in bed. Both eyes are swollen and purplish-black, and Martin tells me this is an almost sure sign of that horrible cancer called neuroblastoma—stage 4, or widely metastatic. Audrey's belly sticks out unnaturally, and I can easily palpate the hard, irregular liver edge well below her ribcage.

Martin has arranged a skeletal survey on the way between clinic and ward, and the radiologist goes over it with us. "See here, and here," she points to spots in her spine, arms and legs where cancer cells have disrupted the normal contour. "Classic appearance, I'm sorry to say. And look at her abdomen, over her left kidney. All those spots of calcification—typical neuroblastoma. What does her bone marrow show?"

"We're about to find out," Martin says. Twenty minutes later, Audrey's nurse has everything ready for me to start an I.V. Her arms are spindly, making it easy to locate veins in her hand. I slide the needle in and hook up the catheter to a bottle of saline. Audrey stares up at me, terrified but barely whimpering.

"A milligram of morphine should do to sedate her," Martin says. "Give it slow and we'll see." Within minutes, she is sound asleep, and we roll her over to get at her posterior iliac crests. "Best place to get marrow samples in children, John. See how the crest sticks out, just under the skin. Good one for your first."

I pull on the powdered rubber gloves the nurse proffers, and Martin hands me the hollow bone marrow needle, attached to the largest syringe I have ever seen—I read off 35 milliliters on the side—and a much smaller one of local anesthetic.

"She'll struggle a bit," he warns the nurse. "Especially when he's tugging out the marrow sample. Well nigh impossible to numb it completely."

Sure enough, as I feel my way with anesthetic under the crest of the bone into where I think the marrow must be, then pull back with the larger syringe, the little girl moans and jerks in her nurse's arms.

"Good sign you're in the right place," Martin murmurs.

Small drops of blood collect in the bottom of the syringe. "Keep pulling. It can be hard to prize marrow fragments loose from the bone. Okay, should be enough, quick, squirt it into these tubes before it clots and you can't use it."

The pathologist calls me early next morning. "That sample you sent me, it's neuroblastoma all right. Clumps of cancer cells all over. I'll send you a slide so you can see for yourself."

It only remains to run the test of Audrey's urine that shows the presence of excessive V.M.A. and H.V.A.—vanillylmandelic and homovanillic acids—that are produced by cancers like neuroblastoma. Two days later we get this final confirmation: both levels are sky-high.

"Big help to have these," Martin says. "We can follow them while we're treating her. If it's working they will fall back towards normal levels."

He takes me with him when he goes to meet her parents. There is a small sitting room next to the ward, with sofa, comfy chairs, and a window looking out on the back garden. I notice for the first time the neat rows of vegetables.

"This is the hardest part, John."

He ushers Audrey's Mom and Dad and nurse in, waits long moments while they settle. Their eyes are filled with fear. Maybe the news won't come as too big a surprise. Martin's voice when he speaks is gentle, his sentences short and clear.

"I'm very sorry, the news isn't good. Audrey has a tumor. A kind of cancer." He pauses. "The technical name is neuroblastoma. It started out in her tummy—her adrenal glands. But sadly, it's already spread to other parts of her body." Another pause, making sure they are taking everything in. "It's in her bones, and the bone marrow which lies inside them. That's why she's been hurting so much, and getting these high fevers."

The mother stares at him wide-eyed. Dad gazes at the hands in his lap. Both are mute.

"We don't know why this happens. You can be sure of one thing, though, neither of you is to blame."

Mom's tears start to flow; Dad's face stays expressionless. This is the first time in my medical life I have sat in on any such conversation—a senior doctor sitting with the family and telling it straight. Actually using the C-word—cancer—no hiding behind half-truths. And no leaving it to some social worker, worse still, me, to break the news.

Dad looks up finally. "What are you going to do, doctor?"

"Well, we have some new drugs the doctors in London and America are using. Chemicals that kill cancer cells. My colleague here"—Martin glances over his shoulder at me—"has researched the latest information, and we think we should try them with Audrey."

Neither parent can summon up more questions, or they are simply terrified of the answers. Martin sits quietly a few more moments, not wanting to fill the room with more words. As he leaves, he puts a hand on each parent's shoulder in turn.

"Sit a little longer. We'll make sure you're not disturbed."

I reflect on the conversation I just witnessed, especially on the things Martin hadn't said. I have read a lot about the newer drugs given to children with "solid" cancers like Audrey's. Adults with the all too common lung, breast, and prostate cancers never seem to receive chemotherapy, but children with kidney and bone cancers are responding to the same drugs we give adults with leukemia. So their different pathologies may be why they respond better, but that isn't the whole story. Children respond far better than adults to cancers like leukemia and lymphoma—among the commonest in children but far from rare in adults—not least because their young bodies handle these toxic drugs better.

But one thing is clear. Even if children are playing an important role in our learning about chemotherapy for cancer, their responses are rarely much more lasting than in adults. A few months in most cases—something Martin didn't feel ready to point out yet to these distraught parents. I have learned a whole lot in a short time about talking to parents of very sick children, with this experienced and caring man to teach me.

I check with the hospital pharmacist about the drugs we plan to use—vincristine and cyclophosphamide. Neither is new to me, having given plenty of both at Barts. Cyclophosphamide is similar to the nitrogen mustard gas stockpiled for possible chemical warfare during WW II, and vincristine comes from the common Madagascar periwinkle, for centuries a folk remedy for all sorts of ailments. But when I show Martin and Quint the papers about using these drugs for children with neuroblastoma, they tell me they have absolutely no such experience. They express worries about the many side effects—low blood counts, throwing up, and many others—all known only too well to me. But if everything I read is right, this five-year-old girl will breeze through her chemo, and hopefully start to benefit.

"Well, if we're going to do this, there is no time to waste. We know only too well how quickly these cancers can spread." Quint glances at Martin, then back at me. "But it's up to you, John. You have all the experience. Good luck."

I go back to the medical ward to explain our plan to the parents and staff nurse in charge. Mom and Dad have somewhat recovered from their initial shock, and eager to hear that we have treatment to offer Audrey. The nurse walks me to the door.

"We haven't ever given this chemotherapy to children we see here with cancer, John. But it sounds like you think it can help Audrey. And you're pretty used to these drugs, so you've got lots to teach us. I'm really happy you're here."

I feel a blush rising up my neck into my cheeks. "Well, thanks. I didn't want to get their hopes up too much, though. I've only ever treated adults myself, so this is brand new territory, and we'll be very much feeling our way."

"Well, good luck!"

As I carry my two syringes of chemo back to Audrey's bedside, I wonder briefly what Sister Kenton's response would have been to this very junior doctor taking it upon himself to administer such experimental therapy. Her mother is asleep in the chair that doubles as a bed. Dad has gone back to work at the local fish processing plant, although I cannot imagine him pulling his full weight. Is there such a thing as compassionate leave for parents in this situation? The I.V. is working fine, so I don't have to put Audrey through that again. I am beginning to take pride in my ability to locate tiny veins in small children without repeated poking. Hardly brain surgery, but a vital skill if I am going to make a career of this. Her mother holds her other hand while I push the needle of each syringe into the tubing, watch the contents slip easily into her bloodstream. The very first child I have ever given anti-cancer drugs. How many others will there be in my future?

"That's all there is to it, Mom. Now we sit back and see how Audrey does over the next several days. With any luck, she'll be feeling a lot better soon. Her temp should come down and she'll stop hurting so much. Then we can give her a second dose next week at this time. And we'll continue her pain medicine as long as she needs it."

But I am unprepared for just how quickly we see results. Next morning, Audrey is sitting up and chatting to Mom, who looks delighted. The little girl's blond hair and pallor give her a frail look, but her response to today's exam belies this. I put her arms and legs through their full range of movement, and she goes along with scarcely a moan. I'm used to seeing younger adults with leukemia respond in a week or two, but this is well nigh miraculous. Another lesson learned: children may get sick quick, but they bounce back just as fast.

"Thank you, doctor. Thank you for giving us back our little one." There are tears once more in Mom's eyes, and I feel my own throat thicken. I distract myself by checking Audrey's I.V. is running okay, then glance back up at her mother.

"Well, I'm pleased to see how quickly she's improving. We're going to keep these fluids running a few days—she needs a lot with this chemotherapy. And she'll probably feel sick to her stomach, not want to eat much."

By the time Audrey's second dose is due, she is up to the bathroom on her own, even making it to the playroom. Apart from mild nausea, she has had no apparent ill effects. Treating my very first child with cancer is proving gratifying indeed. Can I really make a career of this?

"Maybe she could go home and come to outpatients for the next two doses," I suggest to Quint when he joins me. "I could come and give her the drugs, if you agree."

I sense he would not want to be left with that task, and truth to tell, I want to be the one directly responsible for working such apparent magic. After the fourth week, Audrey runs up to me in clinic with a big hug of greeting. When I examine her, I find no trace of the monster that had laid her so low only a month before. None of us have tried to tell Audrey anything about what had struck her down, but she seems to have a blind acceptance of how her life is unfolding. Perhaps this is how children deal with things quite beyond their control.

"We need to stop treatment for a few weeks, let her blood counts recover before we start the next course." I tell Mom. "All the signs are good, but it's best you keep her out of school for the moment, because she could easily pick up nasty bugs. Other than that, she's a normal little girl."

"We'd planned our holidays before Audrey got sick, doctor. We want to take her and her brother down to their cousins in Bournemouth next week. Do you think we can go ahead?"

"That's the very best thing for all of you. I can't imagine your husband is finding it easy to work right now, anyway. And the timing is good, because she won't be missing any treatments. Watch the other children for any infections, and if Audrey should get sick, check into the local hospital and they can phone us. I'll give you a letter for them."

We continue Audrey's treatment throughout the summer and well into the autumn. By the end of seven months, she still shows no sign of the cancer, and her bones look back to normal on X-ray. Then late in November I get a call from Mom.

"She's running a temperature, doctor. And limping on her right leg. She's . . . just not herself."

I had been dreading this moment, knowing it was almost inevitable.

"Perhaps it's just an infection, doctor." I can hear the tears in her voice down the phone.

"Let's hope so." Who am I kidding? "I think we should see her right away, though."

Rosemary calls me an hour later. "Audrey's here, John. I've got some help today, so I can stay with her." And with me, too, I catch myself thinking. I'm going to want someone holding my hand, too.

The telltale signs are all too clear. Audrey lies quietly on the exam table, legs tucked up as though trying to keep them halfway comfy. Although she's running a fever of 101, there's no sign of infection. I feel the hardness of her liver again, and her bones show the ragged moth-eaten appearance on X-ray I have come to recognize. Leaving Radiology, I head straight for the bathroom, praying no one will be there, and lean over the basin in tears. When I get back, Quint is in the clinic office. I feel a swell of relief as he closes the door.

"Rosemary phoned me, John, thought you might want a bit of help here. What do the X-rays show?"

"Much the same as when she first got sick. Just eight months ago."

"You're pretty attached to her, aren't you?"

"They told me in med school not to let that happen. Keep your professional distance was the message."

"Easy to say. It doesn't always work that way, especially with children."

"I'm not sure I'm cut out for this kind of work."

"That's where you're wrong, John. It's the doctors who try to bottle up their feelings, keep that distance, who get into trouble down the road."

I am on the point of losing it again. Quint maybe senses this and promptly becomes matter-of-fact. "I'll go and talk to Audrey's mother. From what you've told me, that drug protocol you used is the best we've got. D'you think there's anything else we should try?"

I pause, sensing Quint will go along with whatever I say, and deeply gratified he is seeking my advice. But all it had taken was a careful perusal of the most recent research papers. By far the hardest part—telling these parents—I am gladly handing over to him. My mind fills with images of all those grown-ups I looked after, who died miserable deaths despite last-ditch therapies—mostly in the accustomed conspiracy of silence. I answer Quint's query, knowing I'm about to seal Audrey's fate.

"At Barts, they were trying out several new drugs on patients whose leukemia had relapsed—more than once. But we used the tried and tested drugs upfront, so the outcome was always the same. A few short-lived responses, but mostly with even more severe side effects. I just don't want to put her through that."

Quint guides the parents to our small sitting room to talk, silently indicating to me to join them while Rosemary tends to Audrey. He starts in without preamble.

"Mr. and Mrs. Saunders, I'm sorry to say I have bad news. Audrey's illness has come back—in full force. The chemotherapy we've been using has simply stopped working. We've done some careful research, and know that this was the only effective therapy available. It's my sad duty to tell you she will not be with us for very long."

Mom crumples in her chair, Dad kneeling down to wrap his arms about her. We sit in a silence broken only by sobs. This time, though, Quint makes no move to go. After long minutes, Mom looks up.

"Is there nothing else, doctor? Nothing we can do?"

"We can make Audrey comfy, so that she won't hurt any more. That we can surely do. We have a room set aside—a private one. You can stay with her all the time."

Neither parent has anything more to say. Audrey lives on for two weeks. Her tummy and bones pains are back, and Quint and Martin let me manage that, too. I explain to her nurses, then her parents, the importance of giving regular pain meds, not waiting until she is hurting again. Fearing their reaction, and my own inexperience, I don't tell her parents we are using morphine—something I've never given to children. But I find small doses prove quickly effective, especially as the little girl is eating next to nothing. I have an inkling the opiate is shortening Audrey's time with us, but no one queries it. Both parents and staff are relieved to see her relaxed and comfy.

The same couple of nurses rotate her care in the private room, and I spend time at her bedside each day, mostly in the late afternoon before finishing work. My fellow house officers are glad to leave me in charge. The Jenny Lind is their first exposure to pediatrics, too, apart from brief med student rotations, and they have never seen a child with cancer either, nor been around dying children. The parents hold a bedside vigil between them, seeing sleep as luxury. Audrey herself spends peaceful hours asleep. I sit beside her, wondering just how death will come. Sometimes I listen to her heart and lungs without using a stethoscope. An innocent intimacy between doctor and patient, which perhaps comforts us both: the two-way nurture of touch.

I can find little to say to Audrey's parents, but they seem to appreciate my presence and not look for more. After the first shock has passed, Mom hesitantly poses the question uppermost in my own mind.

"What's going to happen, doctor?"

I pause to gather my thoughts.

"I think it will be quite peaceful. We can give her stronger pain medicines, but I don't think we'll need to. You're doing the right thing to give her anything to eat that she wants, but I don't think she'll recover her appetite. That's okay, not eating is really okay. All she needs is for you to be close." I hesitate, then, "I don't think it will be long. Perhaps a few days."

Just before the end, I get a phone call from her night nurse.

"She's woken up, John. And she's pretty perky. Chatting away to her parents, though I don't think they understand what she's saying. I thought you'd want to know."

Half an hour later, another call. "Can you come? She fell back asleep just as suddenly as she woke up, and I think she's gone. I can't hear a heartbeat."

Audrey's gray stillness tells the story. Mom clutches her cold hand as she cries quietly, while Dad sits expressionless beside her. I go through the motions of checking for breathing and heartbeat, but nobody expects any resuscitative efforts. I feel a telltale fullness in my own throat, offer a prayer of thanks that this first time of witnessing a child's death has at least been peaceful.

Was that eight extra months of life our chemo had enabled worth having—for Audrey and for her parents? Somehow I think they would each offer a resounding yes.

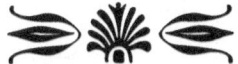

Chapter 4: *LEARNING*

As the year draws on, I grow more and more certain of my chosen path. My weekly essays have me boning up on every aspect of children's health and illness, seeking to master as much as possible of medicine's ever-expanding encyclopedia—narrowing my focus towards children's cancer. But it's my day-and-night encounters with the children themselves that are my real learning. Their irrepressible courage and resilience, their sense of wonder and creativity, are more than a match for the limitations illness lays upon them. I am falling unreservedly for every one of them, and growing in self-confidence in the care I can offer.

Quint runs a special clinic for children with both C.F. and C.P.—cerebral palsy—some of whom have spina bifida, too. I am familiar by now with C.F., but we don't see many children with C.P. on the wards. Before the clinic starts, Quint gives us a rundown.

"To put it simply, cerebral palsy refers to conditions causing limited use and control of a child's muscles," Quint tells me. "Sight and hearing are often limited, as well as swallowing. There are many causes—prematurity, maternal infections in pregnancy, genetic aberrations—but most often we never know the reason. Sadly, many children have severe damage to their brains and not much intellectual function. Many don't live very long, or are placed in long term care facilities. We see just the ones here we feel we can help—which is the minority."

He pauses for my questions, but I am silenced.

"Don't confuse C.P. with spina bifida, though the two can certainly overlap," he goes on. "We see a good number of these children, too. With spina bifida, part of the back of the brain and spine doesn't close over properly in Mom's womb. We don't know why, but it's unfortunately quite common. Most of these children have normal intelligence, though, I'm glad to say. Their problems are mostly muscle weakness, spasticity, and poor coordination. That's where our physiotherapist, Joan, comes in. You'll meet her later."

I tag along as Quint and Joan see the children together. She seems to know everything about their complex anatomy and physiology. The first patient, a ten-year-old, is in a wheelchair, and has almost no use of his trunk and leg muscles. A long scar runs down his back where his spinal defect had been closed at birth. Joan puts his muscles through their full range of movement to counter their stiffness and push them towards their maximum function. Later on, she shows me how to position a little girl with C.F. so she can drain each segment of her lungs. A far-from-gentle art, this tipping a small child into awkward positions while constantly clapping on her frail chest. But Joan is mainly there to teach the parents, who will be their daughter's lifelong trainers, so I feel privileged to sit in.

Quint suggests all three of us house officers sit for the Diploma of Child Health. The idea of adding more initials to my name appeals, and Stephen and I find our way to the examination rooms in a part of London University I rarely visited. There must be two hundred applicants, with so many Asians and Africans we are in a distinct minority. After all our mentorship, the questions seem quite basic.

"Describe the main features of cystic fibrosis. How would you diagnose it, and manage a child with this condition?" "How would you investigate a four-year-old child with anemia?" "What are the causes and complications of cerebral palsy?"

With half an hour to spare, I spend my time reading over my answers, and quickly realize I have quite an editing job on my hands. I am astounded to see how often I have omitted half a sentence. I remember watching Mummy writing a letter, how she would make minor corrections to every word, and how like hers my own writing has become.

The oral exams take place next morning. We are assigned one long case and several quickies. The hall is full of children of all ages, together with moms and a scattering of dads. My mind goes back to my Finals *viva voce*, and my terror at being confronted with a child—a world away from my present confidence, even excitement. As well as the examiners, there are younger men and women directing the traffic. One leads me to the far end of a row of assorted beds and cots. A girl of about fourteen is seated in a wheelchair, and I take in her short twisted legs and child-size crutches. She looks the spit image of several I have met in Quint's clinic.

"You have forty minutes to complete your history-taking and examination," my guide tells me. "You can ask mother and child anything you wish, making your notes on this clipboard. Be sure to respect privacy when you are carrying out your examination."

She indicates two curtains on rollers behind us. I think back to a Barts student who was assigned a blind woman to examine during Finals. He saw no need to pull the curtains around during his examination. "Because she's blind, sir," was his response when the examiner queried this omission. "It didn't seem to matter." His medical career ended abruptly before it had begun.

There is no extra chair, so I shift her crutches over and make room for myself on the edge of the exam couch. Before I can pick up the clipboard and pull out my pen, the girl starts talking. "My name's Sandra. I'm fourteen and I have spina bifida. I was born with it."

"Well, I'm very pleased to meet you. Have you been here before?"

"Third time. I go to Great Ormond Street for check-ups. Lots of us come here for exams. We get paid five pounds—well, Mom does. And they give us a nice big lunch. I know quite a few others here."

Sandra seems to anticipate my every question, and Mom hardly interrupts as she tells her story. Twenty-five minutes later, I have checked off everything I can think of under *HPC*—history of present condition—and *ROS*—review of systems—as well as learning about her family, friends, and schooling.

"I get picked up in this special van every day. The kids at school are really nice. It took them a bit of time getting used to what I could and couldn't do, but now they help a lot. At lunch and stuff. And they take turns pushing me between classes."

As well as their physical disabilities, many patients in Quint's clinic have learning problems, and are either deaf or blind or both. But some have apparently normal intelligence, although I've never met any as articulate as Sandra.

"Don't you want to see all my operation scars?"

I glance at my watch, and discover I have barely fifteen minutes left for the physical. How to get her up on the table and complete everything in time?

Mom anticipates my problem.

"They usually carry out their exam in Sandra's wheelchair; it's hard getting her onto the couch."

By the time the examiner is pulling back the curtain, Sandra has shown me the long curved scar running down her lower spine where the orthopedic surgeon closed the defect in infancy; her leg braces that counter the tightness of leg joints and muscles; and the scars where they have partly released her contracted Achilles tendons. I have time for a quick listen to her heart and lungs, but Mom whispers I won't have to worry about that.

Sure enough, the examiner quizzes me for a few minutes only on the clinical features and management of spina bifida before leading me to my short cases. We come face-to-face with a toddler with an oxygen mask covering most of his face. As I approach, I'm interrupted by a paroxysm of coughing, and what I can see of the face takes on a dusky hue.

"What do you see?"

"He's hooked up to oxygen, sir. Or she," I add quickly, realizing there is no obvious clue as to gender.

"She. Alison's her name. What else?"

"Alison has a barrel chest, sir."

"Good. Diagnosis?"

"Er, cystic fibrosis."

With a nod to Mom and a brief pat on Alison's head, my examiner leads me to a baby who looks about a month old, wrapped in a blanket, sleeping quietly in Mom's arms.

"This child is six months old. He weighs seven pounds. Comments?"

"He is very small for his age. May I ask what he weighed at birth?"

"Four pounds, two ounces. Possible diagnoses?"

"Prematurity, sir. Or intrauterine growth retardation."

"Thank you."

My examination is at an end. A month later, I receive a letter saying that I've passed, and the same week hear my application for a senior house officer job at G.O.S.—the Hospital for Sick Children, Great Ormond Street—has been accepted. We are off back to London. Both Ruth and I are sorry to be leaving the countryside and our Jenny Lind friends, but she seems to accept that this is the only way for me to advance my career.

G.O.S. is a world leader in diagnosing and treating ill children. It started out as a ten-bed townhouse in the 1700s, so it is even older than the Jenny Lind, although hardly rivaling Barts in age. It's stayed independent of the N.H.S., its financial security dependent on legacies like that of the entire proceeds from J.M. Barrie's Peter Pan, in all its iterations and spin-offs. It stands just off Queen Square, an easy walk for Ruth and me from Russell Square tube station. We stroll through the June sunshine to meet Dr. Archie Norman, one of my two new bosses, a senior consultant and pioneer of care for children with C.F. His tenure here must date back to the fifties. I wonder how he coped with the Great Smog of 1952—an immobile and impenetrable "pea-souper" of coal fumes that accumulated throughout that winter and killed an estimated twelve-thousand Londoners.

We walk from his fifth-floor ward onto the balcony surrounding the hospital, to look out on the whole of London's West End. "The children sleep out every night, whatever the weather. Perfect for asthmatics and cystics," my soon-to-be boss tells us. "They think of it as camping out, sheltered from the rain, even occasional snow, by these awnings above. Spend their nights counting the stars."

Ruth and I buy a small second-floor flat for £4500 in Tufnell Park, a mile north of Kings Cross station, and spend our weekends bargain-hunting for furniture in the Camden Town second-hand shops. I am missing Norfolk's exhilarating sea air as I commute to work on London's crowded tubes and double-decker buses. And being thrust back into the halls of academe evokes memories of my daunting Barts days as student and intern, not helped by the G.O.S.'s overwhelmingly scholarly nature. Everyone bows down to its status as the foremost pediatric research hospital in Europe, perhaps the world. Each consultant's patients suffer from only a handful of specific diseases, or ones so rare nobody else has heard of them, which is precisely why they are here.

Ruth is making noises about going back to work, but she has little pediatric experience, and no desire to return to nursing at Barts, which lies only a mile away. I suspect she had hoped to be pregnant by now, or even a new Mom, but I am secretly relieved. Even though, at twenty-eight, I have come to love being around children, I'm not ready for any of my own. I reflect ruefully that there hasn't been too much danger of it—sex has almost gone out the window. I am often distracted by the nurses I'm around each day, and get the sense the interest is mutual, but so far I've resisted the temptation to take any action. I ponder what attracted me to Ruth in the first place, and realize her Welsh background and her dark pretty looks evoked strong memories in me of Mummy. That, coupled with feelings of lostness and loneliness when I had started out on my first Barts internship.

When I got the letter telling me I had landed one of the coveted positions at G.O.S., there was no mention of who I would work for. At least I am familiar with C.F. and its treatment. My big responsibility before Archie Norman's rounds, conducted in detail three times a week on every patient, is to keep the voluminous packets of X-rays in order, so I can instantly pull up the latest chest film for display. Archie is diminutive and mild, and never mocks me for my stumbling efforts. It makes me all the keener to impress him with my erudition, although I'm usually well wide of the mark, often outshone by one of the senior staff nurses.

My other boss is David Hull, a live wire of a man who attracts quite a different clientele, and his rounds are more intimidating. He moves fast from one patient to another, barking out rapid-fire questions and decisions before darting at lightning pace down the corridors to a succession of wards, where he has been asked to render his opinion on an obscure case. I often lose track of him and his research fellow entourage as I haul my trolley-load of charts and X-rays along behind. Hard to figure out his particular expertise: his patients are mostly referred from other children's hospitals, already subject to extensive work-ups for obscure diseases. There are always visiting specialists—American, Australian, and European—doing research attachments, all dauntingly smart and experienced. G.O.S. is the court of last resort, where final judgments are made about obscure diagnoses, usually with bleak outlooks, and David is among a handful looked to for a final verdict.

I learn a batch of arcane lab tests to order on new patients, but I have little energy for the plethora of accessible library resources. But I am mostly spared from being the bearer of bad tidings to parents. Several of Archie's "cystics" are teenagers, and although not much is said, it becomes pretty clear when the end is near. Most die at home, or in their referral hospital, so I never find out how much they understand as their bodies fail, or hear the conversations held between them and their doctors. And many of David's are infants, never destined for long lives, so their deaths seem less tragic. But he makes a point of talking to their parents himself, together with his social worker, and lets me sit in. He always tells them their child's life, and death, was not in vain: they have helped us understand more about some rare condition, perhaps laid the way for developing new approaches for something hitherto untreatable. This is first and foremost a research hospital, and both parents and referring doctors expect nothing to be spared in uncovering novel treatments.

But what do the children themselves think? I reflect on the knotty ethical issues thrown up by adults making every decision for those unable to make their own. My spell as David's resident offers two gems. First, the inestimable value of setting aside time to talk to parents, helping them come to terms with their child's illness. Second, how much the end can justify the means—that these children's experimental, mostly futile, therapies have added to the store of medical knowledge for future generations. A somehow consoling image is of the healthy children of tomorrow clambering over the fallen bodies of those who have gone before.

Meanwhile, I have more mundane tasks to perform. My first Friday on call, the chief resident lets me know there will be a bevy of children admitted for overnight blood transfusions.

"All thalassemics. Greek Cypriots from Kentish Town or thereabouts. They'll start showing up around five o'clock. Same every Friday—we bring them in overnight once the school week is over, so they don't miss out on their lessons. It can take a whole night and well into Saturday to get the job done." He adds somberly, "We transfuse them pretty much every month just to keep them alive."

I struggle to recall my med school teachings on the subject. These children have inherited a gene named for the Mediterranean Sea, rendering them critically anemic soon after birth. I had glazed over the complex explanations in my genetics textbook, but the word, hemoglobinopathy, has somehow stuck: some genetic defect in these children stops them making healthy hemoglobin in their red blood cells. The constant effort to generate fresh red cells of their own causes their marrow spaces to expand inexorably, leaving many of their bones, especially faces and skulls, hugely deformed. They also get overloaded in a few years with all the iron being released from their transfused red cells, damaging their hearts and livers and hormone-producing glands, so they don't grow well and post-pubertal development is a distinct rarity. The adolescent boys' voices don't break, and the girls rarely develop adult-sized breasts, let alone achieve menarche. Our transfusions may be lengthening their lives, but they are also adding fuel to the flames by pouring on toxic loads of iron.

All in all, a short and not very happy life. But we residents have more immediate reasons for asking why our maker created this particular challenge to humankind. It gets harder and harder to locate a virgin vein so as to get our I.V.'s started. Two of us are on call every weekend, starting Friday evening at five o'clock, and we quickly learn we will be spending our nights hauling I.V. trays from bed to bed, struggling to maintain blood flow down these children's scarred and brittle veins. We even compete over how few we have to start, then restart, before a transfusion is complete—often not before "elevensies" on Saturday morning.

We set up I.V.'s on the youngest first, so the nurses can settle them for bed at a reasonable hour. No mean task, because the children get some relief hanging out with their friends, bemoaning their miseries and taking their minds off the trauma they are facing. I overhear two ten-year-olds comparing numbers of sticks during their last admissions. "He poked me here, then here, then here," says one, pointing out each in turn. "I told him this is my best vein"— indicating an unlikely spot on her left wrist—"but he just wouldn't listen. I'd like to stick it right in *him*, see how *he* likes it."

I resolve to query every patient about favored veins, but even this is hard for the teens, so scarred we can fail to establish any blood flow, even when lucky enough to thread in a 25-gauge catheter. Parents often insist on sitting through the whole ordeal, which piles on the stress for everyone, not least us docs. My spirits, already at nadir this first Friday on-call, plummet at the sight of Ilena's name on my list. At eighteen, she is the oldest of the Cypriot girls, and rumor has it on her last admission she flirted with breaking existing records for the number of I.V.'s restarted. It's already 8:45 when I reach her bedside, so I am astonished to find the children's consultant hematologist, Liz Letsky, here. A vivacious Jewish woman in her mid-thirties, she seems to know her patients' life histories as intimately as their medical ones, but even she isn't known for staying at work this late. Is Ilena's illness finally getting the better of her?

On the contrary, it seems more like a birthday party than a deathbed scene. Ilena and Dr. Liz, along with two other colorfully pajama-ed teenagers, are tucking into chunks of angel cake, iced with lurid pink frosting, and washing it down with what I could swear is hard cider. At the sight of me and my trailing trolley, Ilena clambers off her bed, rises to her full four-feet nine, and greets me with a huge beam.

"Doctor, I am the first!"

"Ilena, I'm very sorry to say you're my last. I got way behind with the little ones. I'm really sorry."

"No, no, doctor. You don't *understand*. I am the *first*!" I realize she's blushing, only deepening the mystery. Spotting her patient's embarrassment, Dr. Liz comes to the rescue.

"John, you are looking at the very first of all my young women patients to *menstruate*. Yes, Ilena has started her periods! Now, isn't that cause for celebration?"

It is my turn to blush.

Swept up in the party spirit, the full significance of what I am witnessing doesn't hit me until I am settling down to sleep, well after midnight. A G.O.S. medical record has been broken: despite all the toxic iron deposited in Ilena's ovaries, the transfusions that have kept her alive have spared a small part of her reproductive capacity. Ilena has become the first in two generations of female thalassemia patients at the hospital to menstruate. Perhaps all our sweat and tears are worth it.

Liz takes me under her wing after that. Something about coming on that intimate scene between those four women, and my own sheepish confusion, seems to have lit a spark. I am instantly drawn to her, even though she treats me more as her son than her junior colleague. She starts taking me to visit patients when I can get away, and also to sit in on the hematology clinic she shares with Roger Hardisty, the hematology professor. He leaves the thalassemia children entirely to Liz, along with other patients referred from distant parts with weird problems with their red cells, white cells, or platelets.

She also has responsibility for the hemophilia patients that we house officers rarely see on the wards. When she hears Ruth is looking for work, she offers her a part-time position taking charge of the fresh-frozen plasma stocks used for their treatment. These children often show up as emergencies after a knee or ankle bleed, or troublesome cuts and scrapes from falls, so Ruth acquires a beeper and gets frequent calls to make a plasma run. The children occasionally get admitted for follow-up treatments, so she becomes a presence on the wards too, and like Liz, she gets to know all the patients and families. I find myself drawn to the sight of my wife back in a nurse's uniform and clearly relishing her work. And we are both delighted to have something in common to talk about at day's end.

It turns out that Prof. Hardisty sees solely children with leukemia, most of them on new drug trials. He is a founder member of a national organization that is gathering these children under one treatment umbrella. This comes at minimal cost to the families, because of funding from Medical Research Council and Leukemia & Lymphoma Society grants, something never offered to cancer patients filling the Barts beds. Maybe it's because the incidence of pediatric cancers is $1/100^{th}$ that of adults, so most pediatricians see only a handful in a lifetime, and mostly refer them double-quick to one of a handful of centers.

I am excited to see so many happy children after encountering only the sickest ones in the wards—those newly diagnosed or battling some awful infection. Worst of all, those at death's door and too ill to die at home. Their luckier buddies in Hardisty's clinic seem like normal children, bar their bald heads, because they are in remission and their treatment has become much less intensive. The young ones scamper about in rambunctious games of hide-and-seek, just like those toddlers awaiting circumcision in Jenny Lind's surgical ward. My third time in Hardisty's clinic, he is writing up his history and physical in a three-old's medical chart, absent-mindedly patting her head while she scrawls with colored pencils her own version of events.

He looks up with a quizzical look. "What are you doing next year?"

A question out of left field. I stare back at him, struggling for an answer. Only two months left of my current job, and I have no set plans. He must have sensed my confusion and fills the awkward moment.

"I've got two research fellowships open. Twelve months, paid by the Leukemia Society. You interested?"

My mind flashes on a chap I had come on sitting on a bed in an isolation room where a child with leukemia lay breathing her last. I knew from his white coat he wasn't the dad, but had felt shy talking to him. He must have been one of these research fellows. At that moment, the exam room door swings open and a short, bustling woman appears.

"Carol, this is . . . what's your name again?" Hardisty has the grace to look apologetic.

"Graham-Pole. John."

"Could you find a few minutes to fill John in on what you do? I might recruit him for next year."

Over a brief Christmas holiday, I read all the relevant articles I can find. There being no office space in our Tufnell Park flat, and only one small bookcase filled with Ruth's books, journal papers overflow across the floor under the sitting room window, along with books borrowed from G.O.S.'s medical library. I have two comprehensive pediatric texts: a battered third edition of Nelson's *Pediatrics* and one edited by two unknown Scotsmen. I think about my doctor-dad's Scottish roots; maybe I will make it across the border one day—they must know a thing or two about sick children up there. I am devouring each new *Journal of Pediatrics, Archives of Disease in Childhood,* and *Yearbook of Pediatrics* for everything written in *our* field (which is how I'm starting to think of it). I also make a couple of brief visits to Lewis's and Blackwell's, London's largest academic bookstores, but fail to uncover any books devoted to children with cancer.

On New Year's Day, 1971, two days after my final ward rounds with Archie and David, I report for duty in Roger's clinic. He greets me along with my new colleague, Richard West, whom I have met at lectures and teaching rounds over the past six months. Richard is several years older and dauntingly bright, and I wonder about keeping pace with him. Carol has already instructed us that our primary jobs are blood drawing, plus bone marrow and lumbar puncture tests whenever due. There are also newly diagnosed children to see on the wards, plus those rushed back in with complications from their intensive chemo protocols.

Meanwhile, two nurses work full-time for Roger, lining up the children for their check-ups. He stays put at his desk writing notes in his neat cursive, then poring over the specially printed protocols outlining the child's particular research protocol. Moms and Dads treat him like God, and I reflect on the miracle of having their precious ones snatched back from the jaws of death—unimaginable a few short years back.

Richard tells me this is a fill-in for him while he is awaiting the fellowship promised to him by the consultant he worked for last year. I am secretly relieved, having started to think of him as a rival in this brand new field, especially since there are still no full-time positions in Britain for child cancer specialists. Roger and a handful of other pathologists are the only experts in Britain developing new treatments for children with leukemia and lymphoma. Roger seems to be a largely self-taught pediatrician, but he is certainly an expert on leukemia. His working day consists of moving from research laboratory to clinic and back, when he is not at get-togethers with his cronies. I have rarely seen him visiting the inpatients, and he never attends the weekly pediatric seminars.

I have been reading up on progress in treating children with leukemia in America; we seem about a decade behind here. I come across the name of Doctor Sidney Farber, who in the 1930's became Boston Children's Hospital's first full-time pathologist. This reclusive man indulged a particular fascination with children who had died from cancer, especially leukemia. Meanwhile, the country's leading pediatricians made their daily rounds of the wards, pronouncing to their staff, and the world at large, on the hopelessness of trying to treat these cases. It was simple cruelty, for child and parent alike, to prolong the agony of such dying. Farber was soon christened "doctor of the dead," because of what the senior pediatric staff thought of his morbid fascination with these fatal diseases.

So it was left to this man, with no formal training in pediatrics, to make the breakthrough. In 1947, he tested the first drug treatment for children with leukemia, showing it worked, at least in a handful of cases and for a few months. Twenty years later, I am taking my own first tentative steps into the mysterious world of pediatric cancer therapy, at a time when these children fall way short of growing to adulthood, and there are no trained pediatric oncologists in Britain, nor a recognized training course. Richard is certainly in the majority, using his leukemia fellowship to fill in time while awaiting a job with definite prospects to get his research teeth into. So, unspoken and unwritten though it may be, it is accepted by our country's government, pediatricians, and parents, that a handful of largely lab-based pathologists plan the treatment protocols and write the prescriptions.

So what does this make me? Do I really want to carve out a career treating children with cancer? With only the sketchiest medical school training in pathology—a subject I found largely incomprehensible? When our government has only just got around to appointing the country's first professor of medical oncology? With grown-ups with cancer outnumbering children by a hundred to one? I have to hand it to Dr. Farber. Back in 1947, he was not just a visionary, he was a heroic one. He had seen his early missteps—those children he first treated dying with infections before they could benefit from his experiments—as something to learn from. What drove him to keep venturing upstairs to the wards, almost invisible to these children's families, and numbering absolutely no friends among Harvard's distinguished faculty?

It was only a year earlier that the judges in the "Doctor's Trial" (United States of America v. Karl Brandt, et al, October, 1946-August, 1947) had started to deliberate on Nazi personnel's medical experiments. This would lead to adoption of the Nuremberg Code of Ethics, which is at the core of ethical research principles ever since. But when Farber dreamed up his experiments on these doomed children, there was absolutely no law to distinguish legal from illegal, or to clue their families in on what he was doing. The first thing Farber tried was folic acid injections. Did he know that British children had been spreading large dollops of folic acid on their toast, in the form of Marmite yeast extract —*'love it or hate it'*—since as far back as the 1920's? But these folate shots achieved the very opposite of Farber's intent, actually cranking up the leukemia's march to inevitable death—and further inflaming the wrath of Harvard's pediatricians.

Yet far from retreating back to the safety of his basement laboratory, Farber came to a mind-blowingly simple conclusion. What if he could find something which worked exactly the opposite way—and inject that instead? He discovered from an equally reclusive friend that such a substance existed. This man, known to his friends as "Yella" Subbarao, was an Indian doctor who had come to Boston to train in Tropical Health, but could never get a medical license. His very nickname suggests the built-in racism of the time. He had worked as a night porter before landing work as a research chemist, then taken off to a senior position at Lederle Labs after being denied university tenure.

Subbarao supplied his friend, Sidney Farber, with a package of a molecule he had synthesized from scratch. He claimed it could totally block the action of folic acid in the human body. In September, 1947, Farber started injecting arbitrary doses of this substance into two-year-old Robert Sandler, who had fallen ill with leukemia three weeks earlier and was close to death. It had absolutely no effect on the child's downhill course. But three days after Christmas, Subbarao sent a slightly different form of this anti-folic acid substance, which Farber again administered to Robert. Two months passed, and all signs of leukemia vanished. This lonely pathologist's vision had fired the very first volley in the chemical battle against cancer.

Brits sometimes laugh at Americans for chasing after pipe dreams as if they were going to transform the world. We may be loath to admit it, but taking crazy risks sometimes pays off. As I learn about this medical tipping-point twenty years on, my excitement gathers force. The torrent of papers on treating children with cancer pouring forth in the past two decades almost all come from American pediatricians, who are dedicating themselves to treating children with all sorts of cancers, not just leukemia. So am I ready for some pipe dreams of my own? Is it time for Britain to start catching up by training a few pediatric oncologists—and why can't I be one of them? Maybe it's a good thing I am disinclined to spend my days poring over a microscope in some dusty path lab, would far prefer to spend it staying abreast of everything known about treating these dreadful diseases, and learning how to give my very best care to their sufferers.

I knuckle down with renewed zest. We spend early mornings checking on our inpatient children, meeting with residents and nurses, and ordering the chemotherapy for those newly diagnosed. Three days a week, I am in Roger's clinic, getting to know other children and their parents, then working through the queue awaiting blood tests, bone marrow tests, and their next chemo shot. I become adept at finger pricking to get the necessary blood sample—not easy on a squirming child with a squeamish mom. Building on tips left by our predecessor, I string together a rote of sequential steps:

Get good grasp of sweaty hand;
Unwind tightly clenched middle finger;
Clean off sweat, dirt, and other ickies;
Jab swiftly with lancet so blood flows free;
Massage firmly onto your glass slide before it clots;
Have patient hold cotton ball on wound to keep them busy;
Keep up distracting patter throughout, for everyone's sake including yours.

Then the fun begins. First, spread both thin and thick smears of blood onto a glass microscope slide with a separate "spreader" slide, at just the right angle, speed, and firmness to draw it out by capillary action. Squirt on the required drops of Wright's stain, waving it back and forth like a miniature Union Jack to air-dry. A well-made slide can be a beauty to behold, a lousy one total torment. Last, carefully check the child's name before penciling it onto the frosted end of the slide. Heaven forbid you forget that—or, worse, get it wrong. As far as I know, I never make such a mistake, all too aware of the repercussions from scribbling the wrong name on a slide.

Then on to the microscope. Richard and I had done a fast refresher course before our first clinic, casting our minds back to second-year med school physiology, familiarizing ourselves with the wondrous diversity of white blood cells. Red blood cells hold little interest for us—machines count their numbers and hemoglobin levels, forewarn us of anemia, even estimate their size, color and shape. The lab techs comment on any microcytes, acanthocytes, spherocytes or schistocytes present, which we take largely on trust. All I know is that red cell size and shape tell something of their overall health and function, but with little apparent impact on the children's feelings of wellbeing or otherwise.

As for the platelets essential to blood clotting, we quickly pick up telltale signs when they are running low, and its significance: most often from too much chemo, but sometimes it is the first sign of a relapse of the leukemia. But the white cells are what hold our attention, as we check off "differentials"—the proportions of neutrophils, lymphocytes, eosinophils and monocytes, with the odd basophil thrown in. A good supply of neutrophils means we are not overdosing the chemo and the child is unlikely to fall prey to bacterial infections. The lymphocytes, being the primary catalyst of our immune systems, are often lowered by the immune-suppressing effects of most chemo drugs, and may necessitate a small cut-back in dosage. An excess of eosinophils and basophils means a possible allergic reaction to something, which we might see in the child him- or herself.

Our more challenging tasks are bone marrow exams and lumbar punctures. It turns out the blood counts give us limited information and only betray a relapse when it is well advanced. Every blood cell is born in the marrow, so sampling it lets us spot the earliest sign of reseeding with leukemia cells, meaning the treatment has failed the patient (*not* that the patient has failed the chemo). So Hardisty's protocols call for checking the marrow monthly early on in treatment, plus extra ones when blood counts fall too low or there are suspicious cells on our blood slides.

Lumbar punctures—L.P.'s—are routine, too, when we add anti-leukemia drugs directly into the child's spinal fluid, once we have a sample to test for lurking cancer cells. When you inject chemo into the bloodstream, it may do its job of cleaning out every tissue and organ where cancer cells can lurk, but the drugs stop short of the brain. The existence of this "blood-brain barrier" between blood and cerebrospinal fluid (C.S.F.) has been known since the turn of the twentieth century, but it gained special significance when children with leukemia in apparent complete remission started showing up with severe headaches and vomiting—clear signs of a pressure build-up inside the head. An ophthalmoscope exam would often show swollen optic discs—papilledema—and an L.P. reveals nests of leukemia cells in the C.S.F. trying to escape detection.

It has been ten years since childhood leukemia pioneer, Don Pinkel at St Jude's hospital in Memphis, dreamed up the idea of injecting Farber's anti-leukemia drug, methotrexate, straight into an affected child's spinal fluid. He had no idea of a safe, let alone effective, dose, but twenty-four hours after his first injection, the child who had been gagging and screaming from a violent headache was back playing. As with so much of cancer therapy, Pinkel had to guess not only the optimal dosage, but how often to repeat it. He settled on a short series of weekly intrathecal (into the spinal fluid) shots, and found the leukemia cells disappearing from the C.S.F. without trace. He would have liked to give them more often, but a spinal tap can be as painful as a bone marrow aspiration. After a three-year-old experiences an L.P., she knows exactly what she is in for, and will put up the kind of fight that takes two or three nurses to overcome. Holding a squirming body in precisely the right position to guide the needle into the precise space between those titchy spinal bodies is a hard-learned part of the whole procedure.

Blood collections, bone marrows, L.P.'s, and making microscopic stains for interpretation, are not my only duties. Richard and I are in charge of all protocol orders, then setting up I.V.'s to administer them. Shades of Friday nights among the thalassemics haunt me. I am already handy at snagging a shimmying vein on the back of a wiggling hand, but Roger's "blood clinics" are something else again. I must learn the harsh lesson that the end justifies the means, if I can forestall later and worse suffering. But this is a prescription beyond a young child's capacity to understand, so I must commit my assaults on these little bodies as fast, as skillfully, and as tenderly as I can.

Somehow the children find it in themselves to forgive and mercifully to forget. It is not just that they are robust, they are miraculously tough. They seem to know instinctively that wailing and howling through their suffering helps them through, and their sweet-as-nuts funniness and spontaneous play never utterly desert them. So gradually and painfully, they become my mentors in finding the joy and humor in even the most desperate moments.

Early on, Richard and I rarely have a chance to sit in with Roger, but by the second half of the year, we are getting slicker at our own examining and dispensing duties, so we can spend more time with him. He always welcomes us, knowing if we have time to sit in we must be caught up on any backlog and eager to grab a few minutes of mentorship. During one such lull, I introduce myself to a girl of about fourteen, apparently in robust health and chatting cheekily to Roger, who seems delighted at her grown-up banter. Without preamble, she sweeps me into their conversation.

"I'm Helen. What's your name?"

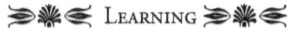

"Hallo, Helen. I'm Dr. Graham-Pole. John."

"Are you a leukemia doctor, too, then?"

"Well, er, I'm hoping to be."

"So you work for the Professor, do you? A trainee?"

"Yes, that's it."

Helen has my attention. I am trying in the worst way to weave through her quick-fire questions without putting my foot in it. I assume she has leukemia, or what is she doing here? But I know I have never had to start an I.V. on her, and she shows none of the telltale signs of the heavy chemo consumer. She even has a head of short dark curls.

"So you like working here, do you?"

"Well, I'm learning a great deal."

"Do you do the bone marrows and stuff?"

"Er, yes."

"Are you good at it?"

"Well, I've had a lot of practice."

Out of the corner of my eye I see Roger trying not to chuckle, while making no attempt to come to my aid. Mom, meanwhile, looks as if she is used to these exchanges and sees no reason to stop her daughter's flow.

"That's good, 'cos I'm due my six-monthly marrow check."

So this is what she's leading up to.

"Oh, so that's why we haven't met before? You don't have shots anymore? Just the odd bone marrow check-up?"

"Yup. It's been seven years. I'm trying to get the prof to stop my treatments. I only have to take a couple of pills every day, anyway, but it's a pain."

Helen hardly flinches as I inject the lidocaine around the iliac crest at the back of her right hip, wait the standard three minutes as it takes effect, then insert my huge trocar and cannula through the track and push down into her child-bones. I feel, rather than hear, the crunch of sharp metal penetrating bone surface, at once start sucking out enough marrow blood for my microscope sample. As always, it comes in a series of drips into my syringe, and invokes an involuntary flinch from the child on the other end. But no murmur.

"Nice job, doc. Hardly felt a thing," is her only comment.

"Wish they were all that easy, Helen. Maybe you could be my assistant, help talk the younger ones through."

"Does it pay well?"

We both giggle. This is why I am doing this job. For these moments, for these children. All of them, even if most are not as obliging as Helen. Back in the clinic, once I have gazed down my microscope at a multiplicity of beautifully maturing cells, I pose the question to Roger that is uppermost in my mind.

"When will you stop her chemo?"

He swivels his chair toward me. "How is her marrow?'

"Healthy as yours or mine. Maybe more so."

"Well, I've never stopped *anyone's* treatment. Our protocols don't really allow for that possibility." He pauses. "But there's nothing to say we can't. I'll check with my colleagues, see if they have any seven-year survivors."

I don't see Helen again before our year finishes. But Roger tells me during my final clinic that he had stopped her chemo that very clinic day.

"It turns out there's a handful of children on this protocol that we're thinking of taking off therapy."

"So how's Helen doing?" I realize I am almost frightened to ask.

"Oh, fine. It's early days, but I've been looking at some of the St. Jude's data. They're beginning to include regular doses of intrathecal methotrexate in their protocols, to prevent central nervous system relapse. They call it 'total therapy.' And also trying to decide how much overall chemo is enough—Pinkel's people suggest maybe three years, but five years seems safer. Anyway, about a third are finishing treatment altogether, and showing no sign of relapse. Keep your fingers crossed—we might have a few of these ourselves."

My fellowship year is nearing its end, and I am back to wondering what next. Eighteen months at G.O.S. has given me a wealth of experience, but I need a registrar training post to ready me fully to become a consultant pediatrician. And it remains a huge uncertainty whether one will ever be available that will let me focus, entirely or even part-time, on caring for children with cancer. I spot an advertisement for two registrar positions at the University of Glasgow, working for Professor Hutchison, famous for his much-reprinted *Textbook of Child Health*.

The whole thing proves easy. Ruth and I make the all-expenses-paid trip by train from Kings Cross, excited to explore a part of the world quite unknown to us. After a night in a hotel in Glasgow's Sauchiehall Street, we sit down for lunch with the professor. He seems delighted at my credentials, tickled by my B.B.C. accent, and impressed I already have a journal publication out and another on the way.

We arrive to start work in the gathering dusk of New Year's Day, 1972, our aging Hillman Imp car barely making it the three-hundred-plus miles between our Islington flat and the Royal Hospital for Sick Children, Yorkhill. We know accommodation awaits us on the premises, but we might have landed on Jupiter for any sign of human life. We gather some ill-assorted nourishment at a convenience store run by an aging Pakistani: two enormous baking potatoes, a cabbage, a packet of oatcakes, a tin of Carnation milk, and another tin bearing a picture of curried pilchards (sardines). I quiz the shopkeeper as I pay for our purchases, while Ruth goes in search of other treasures.

"Will the other shops be open tomorrow?"

"Not yet, good seer." A smiling bow.

"Not on a Tuesday? I mean, in the main street—Argyle Street, is it? Won't they be open for business?"

"Noo, sir. Understand, please, not tomorrow."

"Wednesday, perhaps?"

Another beam and bow, as if in apology for the worshipful company of Glasgow's butchers, grocers, and candlestick makers.

"No, seer, not then."

"So—when?"

He starts to count on his fingers, muttering under his breath, finally beams once more.

"Saturday. Monday, perhaps. It iss Hogmanay, sir."

"What's that?"

"Hogmanay, my good seer. Celebrations! Four day. Five, maybe it could be. We are only shop open this week."

"Hogmanay" is beyond me to spell, let alone decipher. We thank him and make it back uphill to the hospital, where a janitor is dozing at his desk. He conducts us to the doctors' quarters, a grey concrete building set apart from the hospital by pastureland coated with a rime of recent snow. He switches on a light inside the front door.

"On your reet, sir, noomber five. Och, ye'll be comfy enough heer." He unwinds two keys off a hefty keychain from his coat pocket. "One for the missus and one for thissen."

With a brief grunt, he disappears into the gloom. We are more than ready to tackle the pilchards, potatoes and cabbage, but Ruth puts the potatoes aside against the prospect of a week of scarcity. Inspection of the kitchen of our new quarters unearths several half-consumed packets of tea and sugar lumps, and an almost empty salt shaker. But curried pilchards and cabbage, washed down with strong tea, prove a filling combination. I have no thirst for anything stronger, but am craving my first Player's Light of 1972. The night before, we had broken our journey for a New Year's Eve party at sister Mary's home in Yorkshire. Having indulged in a skinful of beer and two packs of cigarettes, I had woken with a hellacious hangover and a firm resolve to finally kick the smoking habit. Ruth, far more abstemious on the alcohol, has no such intention, and had spotted a half-carton of Rothman's at the corner store to supplement her dwindling ciggie supply.

I remove myself from the tempting aroma of tobacco smoke, throw on my overcoat against the chill, and go exploring. The hospital complex is perched on Yorkhill, a steep quarter-mile climb from town in a predominantly working-class Catholic neighborhood, with few owning cars and birth control a mortal sin. I picture exhausted multiparous mothers traipsing up the hill, bearing one or even two bairns-in-arms, with several more straggling along in their wake. I make my hesitant way to the closest building, topped by an illuminated sign, "Accident & Emergency." Apt enough, given the uphill struggle to get here. The atmosphere is still, although it is early evening. A smartly dressed fifty-ish staff nurse greets me.

"Canna help yeh?"

After the polished accents of G.O.S. nurses, her Glaswegian brogue takes me aback. Just as when I first encountered the Yorkshire dialect as a teenager, I am self-conscious about my own clipped B.B.C.

"Er, I'm one of the new doctors here. I just arrived, and was sort of poking around."

"Och, weel, we're surely glad to see yeh. I dinna catch the name?"

"John. John Graham-Pole."

"Graham. That's a Scootish name. What's the oother bit?"

"Yes, my father was Scots. But some generations ago, the family linked the names of 'Graham' and 'Pole' together, and it sort of stuck."

I suspect she is as confused as I was when I first heard this weird explanation. I have always been embarrassed over my double-barreled surname, associating it with upwards mobility towards "poshness" among the middle classes.

"Och, a sassenach thing, neh doot. We Scots keep things simple. All Mac-something or anither—wi' the odd Campbell thrown in. Dora, by the way, tha's ma name. Dora MacLellan. I'll be glad to show you aroond. Tis a wee quiet night so far."

As we walk down a line of cubicles, where two or three young ones and their moms are being attended to, I quiz Dora about Hogmanay.

"Och, it's our big New Year's Eve celebration! Only us workers aren't oot at the parties. And it goes on a long way after—nae a body goos back to work until the fifth day of the year that doesn't need to. Longer this year, wi' the weekend. Street parties, moostly, even when the weather is fierce. Keeping warm wi' anither wee dram!"

"So we won't find any grocery shops open until then?"

"Just the Paki stores. Yeh canna get fresh meat nor fish for love nor money. But there's the cafeteria—that's your best bet. D'ya have any bairns thissen?"

"No. Not yet." I smile to hide my embarrassment. Ruth has had three miscarriages in five years, so we have almost given up on starting a family.

"D'yeh ken who'll yeh be working for?"

"Yes, Professor Hutchison."

"Och, the Proofessor." I hear the capitalizing of his name, the respect in her voice. "He runs this place, trained all the dooctors. A fine man, he is."

"Yes, we came for an interview in November. He seemed a very nice chap."

"Did he take yeh on the Haggis Hunt?"

"Ah, yes. He had me on that one."

"Aye, it's a favorite trick aroon' these parts, whenever we have sassenachs come visit us."

Professor Hutchison, known far and wide as Hutch, had indeed told me the story of venturing forth on "braw neets when the mist is o'er the moor," in Robbie Burns's words, to shoot down haggis as though they were grouse the beaters had put up for our diversion. To much laughter from all in earshot, he had finally explained that haggis is actually a savory pudding of sheep's "pluck" (heart, liver, and lungs), minced with onion and oatmeal, simmered for hours in the animal's stomach and served up with boiled "neeps and tatties" (turnip and potato), then washed down "wi' a dram o' the best malt Scotch." It sounded revolting to my sassenach palette, but I had kept the thought to myself.

I soon discover my fellow registrars were all born and raised in the West of Scotland, all went through Glasgow University's medical school, and had all had internships at the Children's Hospital. So they are thoroughly indoctrinated with Professor Hutchison's *modus operandi*. He expects every staff member on the two professorial wards to attend nine o'clock daily rounds, including the four other consultants. Hutch's control extends to his writing notes in every patient's chart every day.

He is a small man, so it is easy to stay inconspicuous behind hulking Scottish residents, as they hand him charts and are the butt of his probing questions. After the super-specialized atmosphere pervading the G.O.S. wards, I realize I am watching the performance of a dying breed. Hutch knows something, and mostly a good deal, about every medical condition afflicting children. For a generation of Scottish doctors, his textbook has been bible. I know within a few weeks that I will get exactly what I need here—a deep acquaintance with Pediatrics, albeit very much Scottish style.

My colleagues are all here to serve their apprenticeship, then become consultant pediatricians practicing what Hutch preaches in hospitals scattered across the west of Scotland, travelling between two or three cottage hospitals scattered through the surrounding counties of Dunbartonshire, Lanarkshire, and Renfrewshire. I notice Hutch makes briefer visits to the several children with leukemia and other cancers, mostly confined to single rooms, and his notes in their charts are terse. "I agree with Dr. Willoughby's assessment and treatment plan," is his frequent comment.

Of Willoughby himself, the most conspicuous presence is his signature on every hematology report the porters drop into the in-trays. But one lunchtime, once the staff have scattered to other duties, I catch sight of two men donning gowns and masks before entering an isolation room. I quiz the staff nurse about them.

"Och, that's Dr. Willoughby and Dr. Vowels. They do most of the ordering and sich for the wee ones with the cancers." She pauses. "The poor souls, their treatments are worse than their maladies, if yee're askin' me."

I hover outside the room, suddenly shy about gowning up and entering. Strictly speaking, they are Hutch's patients, but essentially cared for by the "Heme team." Hutch had made no mention of Willoughby during my interview, although he knew all about my interest in these children. Most pediatricians still feel the same as this staff nurse—and those 1940's Boston pediatricians—that the treatment is worse than the disease, so barely justifiable.

The two men finally emerge from the isolation room, strip off their gowns and drop them into the special box outside the door. I make my pitch.

"Er, good morning. I'm John Graham-Pole, one of the new registars here. I was wondering if I could make rounds with you?"

The older man smiles broadly. "Oh, we'd be delighted, would we not, Marcus? It would be a treat to have one of Professor Hutchison's doctors join us."

I am astonished to hear this invitation delivered in a plummy English-boarding-school accent, in striking contrast to the prevalent Glasgow dialect. True to his upper-class tones, Dr. Willoughby speaks loudly and distinctly, as though to the whole ward. Only much later do I learn that he too is home-grown, but was packed off by rich parents to prestigious Eton College beside the river Thames at twelve, and that he has put all three of his boys down for his old school before their christenings.

"And this is Marcus Vowels. Perhaps you two have met?"

"No." Marcus is tall and thin, sports a small beard with a shaven upper lip, and offers a brief, shy smile.

"Are you a consultant too?" He looks my age, but better to err on the side of caution.

A further brief smile. "No. I'm here on fellowship. From Sydney."

Another surprise—his accent is broad Oz, quite belying his reticent demeanor.

Dr. Willoughby resumes, "We tend to make rounds about this time. After we've completed the work of the hematology laboratory."

"Perhaps I could join you sometimes? I'm usually free at this time of day."

"We'd be delighted, dear boy."

I manage to join them several times a week after Hutch's rounds. Willoughby is another Hardisty, trained solely in hematopathology, but he spends more time with the patients and families. They may have trouble tuning into his preppy accent and grandiose turns of phrase, but they obviously trust his every word. Rightly so, because I quickly realize he can teach me all I need to become a pediatric oncologist.

Marcus and I have flats in the same building, and Ruth and his wife, Roz, start spending time together. Roz has a part-time job in Willoughby's lab, and encourages Ruth to look for one, too. I put out feelers, and she takes on setting up Glasgow's first organized Hemophilia program. Meanwhile, I keep company most mornings with Marcus, whose job it is to look at unusual blood slides that the technicians set aside. I start to recognize different kinds of anemia, and once more admire the beauty of a well-made blood slide. Dr. Willoughby is obsessive about their quality, spending a good deal of time fussing around the new techs to make sure they meet his ultra-high standards.

But once assigned to my Neonatology rotation, I have little time for anything else. The birth rate is enormous in this Catholic community, and the obstetric and neonatal units are the center for the west of Scotland's high-risk pregnancies, together with emergencies when a premature baby is born unexpectedly in an outlying county. Many of these tinies are judged by the local doctors to be beyond saving, or die before the ambulance makes it to our door. Our consultant neonatologist, Margaret Ferguson, is quick to halt efforts to save a tiny life if she judges it futile. Babies with Down's syndrome, or signs of other severe congenital disorders, are made as comfy as possible and left to fend for themselves. No one seems to have trouble with these judgments, or perhaps parents and staff are both cowed by the authority of the senior doctors. The babies are mostly too weak to suck, and receive water and warmth and little else. This almost always means a quick end, though every so often one simply refuses to die.

Or even two. A year into my Yorkhill tenure, I get a call. It's eleven o'clock on New Years Eve.

"Can yeh come quick, doctor? There's this wee fourteen-year-old lassie, just had twins. A poond or two each, I'm thinkin'. We haven't even weighed 'em yet. She lives with her gran and three other young 'uns in a Gorbals single-end."

I've learned the Glaswegian custom of assessing a patient's living conditions, not just from their address but from how many people share how many rooms. The Gorbals of the seventies is notorious as the worst slum in Glasgow, perhaps Europe—a place where Catholic and Protestant street gangs wage their ancient feuds, while the police steer a wide berth. I do a swift calculation as I scramble into my clothes. Five people in one tenement room—"a single-end"— with one outside privy to be shared with several other families. When I arrive in Accident & Emergency, the duty midwife is lifting the babies onto the scales. They weigh in at 980 and 950 grams respectively. They look identical, but things have happened so fast no one is quite sure how many amniotic sacs, or even if there had been one placenta or two. From what I can fathom, the babies arrived somewhere between grandma phoning for an ambulance and their arrival here.

The midwife swaddles them in blankets in a single crib, their faces almost obscured by masks hooked to oxygen cylinders. Once it is clear that they are gasping at life, I gingerly unwrap them again, take in their dusky, peaked features, panting breaths, swift jumping of heartbeats under translucent chests. I push the tip of my pinky into each puckered mouth, eliciting the feeblest of sucks. This is long before the time such tiny babes would be whisked away to an I.C.U., administered I.V. nutrition and antibiotics, and placed on ventilators. I make a clumsy effort to cover them before they lose more precious body heat, and wonder what next, well aware of Maggie Ferguson's views on extreme preemies from the Gorbals. *Primum non nocere*: first do no harm.

I hear stirring behind me, turn to see Mom curled up on a gurney, staring mutely at her babies as though wondering where they came from. I glance at the chart at the end of the bed, searching for her first name.

"Annie, your boys are both very tiny. You know how far along you were?"

She stays mute.

"Is your grandma around, I wonder?"

"She's doon in Casualty, doctor, givin' the details," the nurse supplies. "Says she's got to be hyin' back home to check on the other young 'uns."

I make a decision. "Annie, I'm going to phone our head doctor, ask her what she advises." I pause, arrested by the fearful face fixed upon me. "We'll keep your little ones comfy, don't you worry."

On the end of the phone, Maggie wastes no time.

"What chance do they have, doctor? You're saying they weigh barely four pounds between them. Those infants just don't make it. Even if they did—either of them—Mom's obviously had no antenatal care, and won't have the faintest clue how to raise them. Best not to do too much, save precious resources." She hesitates, maybe feeling the need to offer reassurance. "Look, I'll see them first thing—if they're still with us—then see what's to be done. Meanwhile, the nurses can try syringing itty-bitty drinks into them, see if they can swallow."

I hang up, turn back to Mom, only to find she's fallen asleep. *Best not to do too much*. I glance at my watch: ten to two. Time to catch a couple of hours.

"Give me a ring first thing," I tell the nurse, "before I go on rounds. Or sooner, of course, if something happens."

I let her know what the boss has instructed about testing them with smidgens of sugar and salt water, and leave the two wee ones gasping behind their outsize masks. Promptly at seven o'clock, the phone pulls me back out of sleep.

"Hi there, doctor," a fresh Glaswegian accent greets me. "Happa Noo Yeer! Your wee twins are gooin' strong. Och, and we've moved them to their oon room in the Kiddies' ward. Mom being just a wee thing herself, it seemed best."

"I'll come right over then. I must say, I never expected them to make it this far."

"Aye, they're toughie wee bairns."

I dash over to the ward, wondering what other surprises await. Is this the point when we step things up, start I.V.'s? The thought of getting even the finest needle into veins the size of grass blades daunts me. I sense someone at my shoulder as I am cautiously unwrapping the swaddling clothes from the babies. I glance around to see Maggie has arrived early for rounds. Maybe she has sensed something unusual in the wind.

"How old are they now?"
"About eight hours since she delivered."
"And how many weeks did O.B. reckon she was?"
"Twenty-eight. Thirty max."
"Stranger things have happened, doctor. Gorbals lass, is she?"
"Yes."

"Must have hardy genes to make it this far. Och, we'd better give them the benefit of the doubt, get I.V.'s started. Would you like a wee bit of help?"

I breathe a sigh of relief. Maggie has a reputation as a dab hand with a needle. I stare in astonishment as she tenderly turns Babe 1's head to one side and sponges antiseptic over his temple.

"Easiest place to find a vein. These preemies' heads are way out of proportion to the rest of them. And you can keep them warmly bundled while you're about it."

She wraps a tourniquet that could fit an adult arm around the infant's scalp, over the barely formed ear. Sure enough, a bluish rising in the flesh under the translucent skin signals the presence of a vein. She places a 25-gauge needle flat to the skin, dips it down a fraction, and is rewarded with a flow of blood back into her syringe. She draws a couple of milliliters before hooking up the intravenous line.

"Get the usual newborn screen on this," she instructs, handing me the sample to dispense into tubes. "And don't waste it—that's half a pint to them." She fixes tape over the business end of the I.V. on the hairless scalp. "See, the temple makes a nice flat surface to rest my needle. Should last a day or two—if he does."

She watches over my shoulder as I tackle Babe 2. I feel a trickle of sweat on the back of my neck, remember to slow down and breathe. Following her example, I am gratified to hit a scalp vein first go. My fingers are sticky and clumsy, but I manage to draw the same two milliliters and fasten the line in place without any fatal jogging. I straighten up and register my aching back from hunching over the crib, make a mental note to sit down next time.

I expect new trouble when I show up for each early-morning ward round, only to be greeted by the boys sleeping peacefully on their sides, one at each end of their crib. Just like how sister Jane and I would sleep top-to-toe as little ones in the same bed on cold winter nights. Very comforting.

The two bairns know no rules bar their own. I only have to start new I.V.'s a couple of times on each: within a week they are swallowing enough from syringes to give them a modicum of nourishment. I watch in fascination as two tiny tongues peek out from birdlike mouths, savoring the sweetness and not wasting a drop. On day seven, I am startled to find Annie leaning over the crib side crooning softly. I tune into the dulcet tone of the melody, maybe an old Scottish lullaby. She had gone home with Gran a few days after she had popped them out, and I hadn't seen her since. Perhaps the staff has warned her away, not wanting her to become too attached.

A nurse has unwrapped the blankets a bit, so Annie can more easily ogle her boys. I stand quietly as she starts to talk to each in turn, feeling guilty at listening in on this private conversation. But her Gorbals vernacular is well nigh impenetrable.

"Will tha luk a tha bairns' fuit . . . tha een." Then as each starts to whimper: "Och, they're greetin' . . . theer, theer, dinnah fash thissen."

I have only a faint notion of what she's telling her twins, though it seems too intimate a moment to interrupt, let alone ask for translation. But it's time to gently let her know I am here.

"I think perhaps they're getting a mite cold, Annie. We must be careful not to chill them. They're not too good at keeping their temps up."

I am unsure if even this short explanation has sunk in, but she offers no protest when I reach down to wrap the blankets back around them. A nurse greets us both.

"Hi there, I'm Eileen, the babies' nurse today. Real champs, they are. We're reet prood of 'em."

"Why are mah bairns greetin'?" Mom asks her, probably more comfy with one of her own. Perhaps she's detected my *sassenach* origins.

"Och, they were maybe a wee bit chilled, hen, like doctor said. See, they're quietin' doon nice noo. Don't goo upsitting yerself, dearie."

Eileen's accent is almost as broad as Annie's, but I figure this is a good time to supplement the "Vocabulary of Robert Burns," a 1935 edition I have borrowed from the local library, and learn a little more of the Glaswegian vernacular, with a local nurse to help me.

"I didn't quite catch what Mom was saying," I tell Eileen, blushing slightly. "I'd like to be able to, you know, understand her a little better."

"Och, she talks the auld Glaswegian, doctor. Let's see . . . 'fuit' are 'feet' and 'een' would be 'eyes.' 'Greetin'—that's 'cryin.'' What else? 'Dinna fash thissen' means 'don't upset yourselves.' Theer, ye'll be catchin' on in noo time."

I am rewarded with a broad grin from Annie, and feel a lump in my throat at connecting across such a divide of language and background.

Next day, I meet with the boys' great-grandma for the first time. She has taken to keeping Annie company on the number seven bus from the Gorbals to the bottom of Yorkhill for daily visits. Their conversation consists mostly of terse grunts from Grannie and minimal responses from Annie. I sense there is little love lost between them, and that they are starting to wonder what will happen should the twins make it out of hospital. No man claiming any link to the boys has been spotted on the unit. Perhaps not surprising, as the social worker's discreet enquiries have elicited that Annie has had a string of short-lived male admirers, any of whom could be dad.

A month after their birth, Annie is yet to name her boys. Perhaps she hasn't wanted to tempt fate as they cling to life. I am sitting beside her as she nurses twin 1 in her arms and cautiously coaxes it with a small bottle of breast milk the nurses have taught her to express. Our brief conversations involve a lot of sign language, and I have come to not expect much more.

"Wa's thee gien name?"

At first, I think she's talking to her baby, as she hasn't lifted her eyes from him. Then she glances shyly towards me.

"What's yer name?"

"You mean my Christian name?"

"Aye."

"John."

"An' yer faither's?"

"Richard."

"Och, thass it. John 'n Richard, I'm namin' 'em."

Two unlikely sassenach names for these dyed-in-the-wool Scots-Irish boys, but I refrain from saying so.

"Annie, I'm honored you should choose our names. Which is John and which is Richard?"

"I dunna. Yeh decide."

Wondering briefly if this falls within the purview of my job description, I lay a hand on the nearest one's head, feeling like a priest performing baptism.

"John." I repeat my little ritual with the second twin. "And Richard."

The lump in my throat is back.

Four weeks later, Annie takes her precious bundles home to her single-end. They top almost four pounds each on the nursery's scales, and she could tuck them both in her purse and sling it over one skinny shoulder. But John and Richard have smiles for all who come to ogle them, and lusty sucks for every ounce of milk on offer. Annie has utterly recovered from her initial shock and is showing herself a devoted mom, even breastfeeding them for short spells. Perhaps her loving touch is the secret to their thriving. Something that would have been denied them in a more high-tech environment. Even Gran has come to terms with these sudden additions to her family. Their unlikely survival has drawn widespread attention, and money and household goods are pouring in. We have set up frequent health visitor checks-ups at home, as well as follow-up in clinic. Annie will be joining the daily hordes of big-bellied women swaying their way up Yorkhill from the Argyle Street bus stop, towing behind them strings of grubby and unwilling children.

Who knows what the future holds, but some higher order has been watching over the twins until now. As Kirkegaard said, life is a mystery to be lived, not a problem to be solved.

Our first year has flown by, and Ruth and I start talking about adopting our own baby. The gynecologist, a tall, spare Scotsman, looks at us dubiously from behind his desk and announces that Ruth's miscarriages are due to something he terms an 'incompetent cervix.'

"Ye see, your cervix opens up too wide to keep the baby inside until it's big enough. There's this fellow over to Edinburgh—and a few down in your neck of the woods—who've tried tying it closed early on, then taking those wee sutures out before the bairn is born. I'm agin' it meself, lass. Go get yourself pregnant, and then we'll see what we can do for ye. Bed rest is the best remedy to my way of thinkin'."

No more pregnancies come our way, perhaps because both of us have once more lost much energy for sex. But my experience with Annie from the Gorbals has stayed with me, and both Ruth and I are increasingly taken with the idea of adopting. Perhaps being new parents will rekindle the spark in our relationship. So after several phone calls, we make our way to the social worker's office attached to the Royal Maternity Hospital in Rottenrow. The plaque above the building's entrance reads, "The Royal Lying-In Hospital and Dispensary, 1834." We have chosen Rottenrow over the more up-to-date University of Glasgow's maternity unit, where wait times for adopting babies are much longer. There is good-natured dispute among Glaswegians about whether the street's name derives from the old Gaelic for "road of the kings" or "infested with rats," referring in very different ways to its 14th-century origins. I favor the latter—the place looks like it hasn't seen any repairs since they laid the foundations.

The social worker expresses delight at having a budding pediatrician and his wife on her list. "Aye, there's many a lassie burdened with an unwanted wee one, who hasn't the means to provide for him. I should have news for yeh by year's end." We can take ourselves off her list any time, but it feels like the die is cast, and as the months pass we start to anticipate that phone call. It comes late in September. Three-month-old Gavin is awaiting adoption, and we are top of the list. The social worker reassures us it is customary for adopting parents to choose their own name, and by the time we arrive at the foster parents' home, we have decided on George. Ruth has brought his crib in our car, but once we have signed the requisite forms, she ends up in the back seat with him in her arms as we head home.

I have taken a week's leave, so we can both get acquainted with our new son, and the next few days pass in domestic bliss. George proves to be a most contented baby, waking for feeding only once through the night, which we take in turns. I love burping him, changing his nappies, and simply cuddling him. Fatherhood is proving all it's cracked up to be, and within the month, we have decided to explore the possibility of adopting a second child.

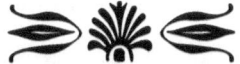

Chapter 5: *CLIMBING*

Dr. Willoughby starts talking to me about a new project. He has installed an American apparatus called a continuous flow cell separator, which occupies pride of place in the lab. It is a giant box on wheels with a stand attached behind, and loops of I.V. tubing disappearing into the business end in front.

"John, I'm most excited about this." His upper-class drawl barely contains his delight. "The procedure is awfully like donating blood, d'you see? Only we have the person's blood run straight through this centrifuge," pointing to a translucent plastic bowl inset into the box. "Then, Bob's your uncle, the blood separates in the most *splendid* way into its component parts. Red cells, plasma, and most especially, the white cells in the middle. The most elegant thing imaginable!" He pauses for my reaction.

"So we can select just the bit we want?"

"Absolutely, dear boy, you've hit the nail on the noggin!" He whirls around and beckons one of the senior techs. "Maggie, be a dear and bring one of your centrifuge tubes, one you've just worked with." He holds up the transparent glass tube she hands him. "You're of course totally familiar with this, John. You see the buffy coat right there, sandwiched between red cells and plasma?"

Sure enough, the narrow white band is unmistakable, lying between a column of red cells at the bottom and the pale yellow plasma on top. Extraordinary I never paid attention to such a commonplace thing.

"Just imagine being able to circulate the whole of a person's blood through this machine over and over again." Dr. Willoughby is almost jumping up and down in his exuberance. "The manufacturers claim you can process ten liters of blood in under four hours. More than twice an adult's blood volume—astounding! We can collect unlimited numbers of healthy white cells to transfuse into our patients in dire need. I haven't found a single paper in the pediatric literature about this—have a hunt around for yourself. Meanwhile, we have a gentleman coming from Houston to demonstrate this whole technology."

I quickly uncover a few American researchers who are using this apparatus to transfuse granulocytes—more correctly, neutrophils—into cancer patients with life-threatening septicemias and other infections. Neutrophils are the white cells at the forefront of our defense against bacterial infections, and chemotherapy often leaves patients temporarily without a neutrophil to their name. But I can find nothing written about doing so with children in the same plight.

I think back to a four-year-old from Ayr, the county town of Ayrshire, who had arrived on our doorstep two weeks earlier. Her pediatrician had correctly diagnosed her leukemia and started treating her, only to watch her quickly succumb to what proved to be *E. Coli* septicemia, an infection from which few severely neutropenic patients recover. We had been standing ready and had filled her full of potent I.V. antibiotics as soon as the ambulance pulled into our A.&E., but she was gone before we could even get her up to the ward. I had been the one to break the news to her parents in the corridor outside. What if we had had time to get one of them onto this cell separator, and transfuse their white cells into their little girl? Might things have turned out differently?

I am catching Willoughby's excitement. He obviously thinks the cell separator offers a chance for some major collaborative work. He knows as well as I do the sacred dictum, "publish or perish!," and is pressing me to make a name for myself in this new line of research. The Texan arrives from Houston the day after my first demonstration. He has stepped right out of "Midnight Cowboy," the film Ruth and I had caught just before leaving London: immaculately pressed sky-blue Levi's set off by a longhorn belt buckle, fringed suede jacket, and snakeskin boots. Willoughby introduces him.

"Ah, hallo, John. This is Mr. Malone. From Houston."

The man wheels about to greet me and flashes a winning beam. "Y'all call me Clint, ya hear! Ah'm mighty pleased to meet you, John."

Willoughby continues, barely concealing a giggle. "I've asked John to take a special interest in our research with the cell separator. He is one of our rising stars in the pediatric world." Clint directs the full glow of his attention on me. It is hard not to step back a foot or two from this full-face confrontation. British conventions of comfortable distance clearly don't apply.

"John, ah'm fixin' to show you ever' little thang y'all need to know."

And there is never any doubt Clint Malone—even his name draws smirks as he introduces himself to all and sundry—knows his stuff. The first day, we gather around the machine—Clint, Mike, myself, and Maggie, the tech Mike has assigned to the task. Our Texan has exchanged his sky-blue Levis for off-white ones, set off by a ten-gallon Cowboy hat, which he makes a big play of doffing each time he is introduced to a lady. At first, I think his Southern drawl must be a put-on, but it never wavers in pitch or tone, if anything becoming more pronounced as he takes his ease with us.

He clearly basks in his expertise, and is a natural teacher. He explains step-by-step the intricacies of how to operate the system, with always the quick inquiry: "How's it comin', guys?" or "Y'all with me on that, good buddy?" At the hands of this unusual mentor, it takes me no time to get over any fear of reproof, still deeply entrenched from my full-time schooling from six to twenty-six. I find myself stopping at each stage to have him run it by me again, all the while scribbling copious notes. Maggie, meanwhile, seems to grasp everything straight off. Even her queries display a technical knowledge I have never acquired—nor had any desire to.

Willoughby stops in at regular intervals, but he is clearly happy leaving things in our hands. For our first "live" experiment, he hands Clint two bags of fairly fresh whole blood to prime the machine. Once the blood is flowing freely into the centrifuge bowl, we lean in as our teacher demonstrates the rapid separation of plasma from red cells. A few minutes later, a narrow, pale band, less that a centimeter across, defines itself between the two other parts of the blood.

"Thar she goes, sure 'nuff." Clint is taking obvious delight in our oohs and aahs. "But jes' you wait until you get the real thang. Them thar white cells ain't near as good as a real fresh donor's."

We have living proof that very Friday, the day before Clint's departure back to Houston. Will, a seven-year-old boy who had gone home last weekend after his first month of chemo for leukemia, ends up back in isolation with a high fever. Twenty-four hours later, the bacteriology lab phones to say *E. Coli* is growing out of his blood culture sample. I approach his parents at Will's bedside, where he is sleeping fretfully. His temperature had peaked half-an-hour earlier at 103.6.

"Mr. and Mrs. MacMahon, Will has a very serious infection in his blood. We are giving him the strongest antibiotics we have, but sometimes that just isn't enough. Have either of you ever been a blood donor?"

"Aye, doctor," Dad answers, "I've gi'en a few pints in me time. I'm O negative—universal donor, they say."

I breathe a sigh of relief; this will make it so much easier. Not only has he been a blood donor but Will is also O positive. Clint has pointed out that matching up A.B.O. blood groups between donor and receiver of a granulocyte transfusion is hugely important, because the system for separating them is far from perfect, and there will be an unavoidable quantity of red cells mixed in with the white ones.

"Well, Mr. MacMahon, I have a proposal for you. Dr. Willoughby and I believe you can be a blood donor for your son. Of your healthy white blood cells, that is, not your red cells. We have a special machine to collect them—without risk to yourself, other than the usual ones with any donor. It's those white cells of yours that can help Will fight back against his infection."

As I speak, I am surreptitiously eying his forearms below his rolled-up shirt sleeves. I fancy it won't be hard getting a good blood flow from this brawny Scot's veins. Four hours later, we're unhooking him from the cell separator, everything having run like clockwork under Clint's watchful eye. We have been checking small samples of the cloudy white concentrate in the bag we will soon be transfusing into Will. A quick estimate on the Coulter counter tells us the bag holds a concentration of white cells more than ten times Mr. MacMahon's normal white blood count.

There is one other essential thing before we can hang the bag—to give it a small dose of radiation to make sure none of dad's lymphocytes become permanently engrafted into his son, which could cause a whole new set of problems. The transfusion takes less than an hour, while I hover at the bedside half-expecting unforeseen calamity. But Will sleeps blissfully through, as Mom checks on her husband to make sure he has suffered no ill effects.

An hour later, the boy's white count has shot up from zero into the thousands. Next morning it is right back down again, but so is his fever—and joy on joy, *E. coli* is no longer growing from his blood. To make doubly sure, we repeat the whole procedure, with the same happy results. A week later, Will's defenses are reasserting themselves, and his white cell count is climbing on its own towards normal. Clint assures me it is safe to use the same healthy donor as many as four times in one week, because human beings regenerate white cells far quicker than we do red cells or platelets. I shake hands with Will's parents as they pack up their belongings to head home.

"I didn't tell you before, but both you and Will were what you might call guinea pigs. It's the first time we've used our machine since it arrived from America. We think Will is the first child in Britain ever to get this treatment."

"Perhaps it's just as well yeh didna' tell us that afore, doctor. We might jest a' got a wee tooch o' cold feet."

"Well, you two will be the first of many. You have every reason to take pride in what you've done for Will. And for many children to come."

A year later, Mike and I pore over our results. Of the ten children with leukemia who have received transfusions of white blood cells from a parent, eight have shown every sign of responding and are doing just great. Only two have died, both of whom had arrived on our doorstep already at death's door with horrible infections. Because our hospital is where doctors throughout the west of Scotland send their tough cases, we are getting increasing numbers of calls. Then a senior registrar puts in a phone call from Newcastle-on-Tyne—so-called Geordie country in north-east England. He arrives in an ambulance four hours later, accompanied by a breathless and frightened teenager on a stretcher.

"We diagnosed acute myeloid leukemia five days ago," my colleague says. "He's got bilateral pneumonia and the lab phoned early today to say they're growing staph aureus from his blood. I didn't want to wait any longer—we had to give him oxygen on the way up. Mom's not an ABO match, and his dad isn't in the picture. But Ryan and I are both O+ve. I'm happy to donate."

Alan, the Newcastle doctor, proves a cheerful companion while he is on the cell separator. Maggie is a dab hand at running things while I am off on other duties, and my main task is starting the I.V.'s, then getting the donor safely off the machine at the end. I'm nervous putting an I.V. into a colleague, my mind thrown back to fumbling attempts at practicing blood draws on fellow Barts students. But all goes well for both patient and donor.

"Did you see the call for papers for the B.P.A. conference next spring?" Alan quizzes me as I pull out his I.V. lines and strap on good-sized bandages. You should present your stuff. It's exciting."

That evening, I find the advertisement calling for papers to present at the British Pediatric Association next April, and put together an abstract describing our first twenty cases. It is to take place in York, so Ruth and I can spend time with my sister, Mary, in nearby Harrogate. This will be my first big presentation, and I feel a mix of excitement and trepidation when my paper is accepted. I spend February and March poring over my notes, reading it aloud every night to make sure I stay inside the permitted twenty minutes.

"Patients received granulocyte transfusions if they had infections associated with severe neutropenia ($\leq 300/mm^3$) not responding to antibiotics after a mean period of 72 hours. . . . The clinical state of the patients was assessed 24 hours and 5 days after transfusion. . . . No control patients were studied for comparison. . . . Student's 't' test was used for statistical analysis . . ."

"Does it sound academic enough?" I quiz Ruth.

"Certainly the kind of thing to put everyone to sleep in the first five minutes."

"Well. I admit it *is* pretty dry stuff. Isn't that what academic papers are about?"

"Will you be okay if I skip the conference and stay with Mary?"

"Fine. I'll certainly be putting you to sleep a few times by the time I've finished polishing it."

The night before my presentation, I anticipate the daunting sight of five-hundred pediatricians gazing at me at the lectern. After a quick dinner with friends from G.O.S. days, I closet myself in my hotel room and take up the five dog-eared pages of my speech. I switch on my portable projector, and scan my life's work for the umpteenth time—a 276-page doctoral dissertation compressed into twenty slides. I have it down word-for-word, but my mind is jumping like washing in a wind storm. I decide to just run it through a couple more times. At 2:40 a.m. I fall into an edgy slumber, replete with dreams of serried ranks in dim lit halls. At breakfast, a paternal hand drops on my shoulder. I twist my head. Dan, our children's surgeon, grins at me. The grin of a troll. He squeezes down on my acromion.

"Ah think I'll gi' tha' wee talk of yoors a miss, Johnnie. I was in the room nex' door, heerd it more than a few times through the early hours. Reckon I could gi' it missen!"

My blush rises from chest to forehead. Why the hell didn't he bang on the wall to shut me up? Did he lose beauty sleep simply so he could make a monkey of me over my eggs and bacon? With a light clap on my scapula he is gone, leaving me to sally forth and wow the august hordes with my erudition and eloquence.

But it goes smoothly enough, and I even leave the requisite time for questions. I'm disconcerted I only get a couple of trivial ones from greybeards in the front row, and one younger chap at the back who takes several minutes to spout his own opinions, with no question attached. Anna Murphy, one of our junior Yorkhill consultants, joins me for coffee.

"Congratulations, young man. You did great."

"Well, it didn't seem to spark much interest."

"Och, not to worry yoursen' aboot that. It probably went over most of their heads. 'Tis important work ye're doing. I hope Hutch can find you a permanent position so yeh don't flee back to London."

Anna's words come back to me when my last year gets under way, and I start wondering if indeed my boss can create a permanent position for me. There is certainly plenty of work to do, now that children with cancer are taking up more and more beds on the wards, and I have succeeded in getting several articles into medical journals. Time to bite the bullet. Hutch's secretary makes me an appointment, and the next day he ushers me into his office after morning rounds.

"What's on your mind, my boy?"

"Well, sir, I've been thinking about next year. I've very much enjoyed my time here, and I feel there are great opportunities."

"That's for sure. And you've done very well."

"Thank you, sir." I hesitate, then plunge on. "Do you think there's a chance of a permanent position for me?"

"Ah, so that's it." He pauses for an ruminative moment. I can almost hear wheels revolving in this canny Scotsman's head. "Well, you certainly deserve the opportunity. And we would love to keep you. I'm going to look into our financial situation very carefully."

Now for the big one. "With that in mind, sir, I feel I need to get a broader vision of the field. There are several pediatric oncology centers in America. I feel it is essential to make a visit, learn firsthand about new research trends. And so on."

I tail off lamely, all too aware of his scrutiny, and of my own boldness. But he surprises me.

"How long are you thinking?"

"Six weeks," I blurt out. "That would give me time to visit Dana Farber, Sloan Memorial in New York, St Jude's . . ."

He cuts me short. The names mean nothing to him. "That's a good proposition. We should be able to find the funds. Look into it, see what it will all add up to."

I can't believe what I am hearing. Is this a done deal? Can I really go mix with the bigwigs in the field, be in on the latest ideas? I decide on six centers, time to meet with the top people, make ward rounds, sit in on teaching sessions, see how they run their clinics, and figure out how to set up my own program. I write letters to Roswell Park in Buffalo, Dana Farber in Boston, Sloan Kettering, Children's Hospital of Philadelphia, MD Anderson in Houston, and—the cream of the crop—St. Jude's Childrens Research Hospital, in Memphis. I get warm letters from all, promising to make my time "richly fulfilling," "a positive interchange of ideas," and "satisfaction guaranteed." I put it in the hands of the Sauchiehall Street travel agent that Hutch's secretary directs me to.

It is quickly clear that entertaining visitors from afar goes with the territory. I am also expected to give at least a couple of talks, so I can fill my new American friends in on "what you Brits are up to." A terrifying prospect, but at least I am no longer a total stranger to public speaking. As I make plans for the trip, Ruth and I are sidelined, much to our delight, by a fresh call from Rottenrow: a little girl awaits us. It is the third week of December, so we'll be celebrating with a very special Christmas present. We are much less prepared this time, so Ruth and I scurry around collecting the necessary paraphernalia. But at least we both feel we know something about raising babies. The social worker has made only one home visit since we adopted George, and must have been satisfied about our suitability for a second child.

Kate, as we christen her, turns out to be a redhead of Scottish-Irish stock, like her brother, and only ten days old. But unlike George, she has a hard time settling into her new home, crying inconsolably every night despite all the tricks we conjure up. George is delighted with his new sister, and insists on helping me with each feed. And I am as besotted with her as with my son. By late January, she is settling in, and we start attending the local Anglican church most Sundays when I am not on call. Both George and Kate sleep peacefully through the service, waking up in time to be passed around over tea and biscuits in the hall.

The services are the same as we sometimes attended back in London.

I don't give much thought to their religious content, but we start making friends with other young parents and a few university folk. A neurologist and his wife invite us to the local curling rink, where there is a crèche for children. Neither of us is much good, but we are assigned to teams each time, and the skips are helpful and supportive. Suddenly, I have a life away from work, and a smile on my face when I hit the front door each evening. Ruth and I are as close as we have been throughout our marriage, and we even start love-making again—something I had come to think was banished to the scrapheap of memory. We are finding lots of new parent stuff to plan and talk about, and even loss of sleep isn't blighting our newfound marital harmony.

I decide to finalize plans for my trip. Ruth assures me she'll be okay coping with both children, and she is getting a good deal of help from two teenage girls from church. I make arrangements for six weeks leave and book my flight to Buffalo, New York, and in no time am scurrying down the ramp at the Buffalo airport. I change my traveler's checks into dollars and grab a taxi to the hotel connected to Roswell Park Institute. I am due for dinner at a downtown restaurant that my host, Arnie Freeman, had identified in a follow-up letter, to which he had attached a dizzying five-day schedule. Warned it would be hot and humid in late August, I change into the lightweight suit I had splashed out on in Glasgow's only trendy men's shop. Arnie is skinny and crew-cut, in shirt sleeves and wrinkled pants stopping two inches above his ankles. He regales me over stiff cocktails with a list of his program's accomplishments and ambitions.

The menu is too huge to take in, so I mimic Arnie's "Hamburger, all the way, but hold the fries, will ya? And a side order of onion rings." I struggle not to blush, avoiding both Arnie's and the waitress's eye, and silently compute the calorie content of French fries and onion rings. Arnie clearly doesn't have a weight problem, but six weeks on an exclusive hamburger diet will leave me panting if I have to chase down a bus. Maybe I'll stick to salads, apparently gratis of the management.

"Caesar, French, Italian, Thousand Island, Roquefort, or Creamy Ranch?"

"Er . . ." What on earth is she talking about? The blush rises once more. Arnie grasps my discomfort and grins broadly.

"He's a limey, babe, just off the boat. They only have one salad dressing over there."

The penny drops. Salad dressing! But how on earth to choose?

"He'll go for the Thousand Island. Me—just oil and vinegar on the side."

I store this away for future use, while Arnie talks up his multi-center consortium to "lick kids' cancer." I thank my stars Roswell isn't one of the places that I will be propounding on how I'm about to do the same. As rounds get under way at eight next morning, Arnie heads off at a dead run, introducing me jauntily to every resident, fellow-in-training, nurse, and ward pharmacist. There are fifteen patients in this dedicated children's cancer ward, mostly confined to single rooms. The staff congregates outside each room as Arnie takes me in for more introductions, mostly to Moms, accompanied by head pats for youngsters and brief joshes with teens. The patients are all on one research protocol or another, with the research fellows current on every aspect, while the residents seem not to know the difference between leukemia and leprosy. But they have a well-honed way of presenting each patient that mostly sees them through.

"Fourteen-year-old Caucasian female, status post-reinduction for ALL, protocol week eight, multiple admits for chemo admin, fever and neutropenia. Current admission precipitated by 36 hours fever and night sweats. P.E. positive for mucositis, grade 3, scalp alopecia, diffuse obesity, facial and truncal acne, grade II striae, loss of muscle bulk in central areas. C.B.C. . . ."

"Hold it right there, Curt. What protocol? What chemo?"

Curt grabs the chart. "Er . . . Prednisone, vincristine, daunomy . . ." He stumbles over an obviously foreign word. Arnie glares.

"These kids are in your hands. You gotta know their therapy, the whole deal. Side effects of dauno?"

"Er . . . mucositis, alopecia, neutropenia . . ."

"Heart failure! Don't you know it's cardiotoxic? What about her cardiac exam?"

Curt looks ready to burst into tears. One of the fellows intervenes. "We'll go over it right after rounds, sir."

Arnie swivels his dirty look towards him, then reverts to a grinning, "You guys . . ."

Teaching pediatrics American style. A million miles from Professor Hutchison's wards at Yorkhill.

The rest of the week passes in a flurry of doctor meetings, research sessions, teaching conferences, and nights spent poring over Arnie's publications. My last night, he hosts a wild party around an industrial-sized barbecue in his backyard. Half the hospital seems to be there, alongside many neighbors. I climb on an early-morning plane to New York City, my hangover trumped by mounting exhilaration. There seem to be no lost causes. If all Americans are as dedicated to saving children's lives, I am with them all the way.

The laconic cabbie warms up when he learns I'm a limey doc, and starts pointing out the sights of Manhattan as we cross the East River and sweep down F.D.R. Drive toward Central Park. My first sight of Memorial Sloan–Kettering Cancer Center, spread across a couple of city blocks, daunts me. "Easy stroll to the park in your lunch hour, grab a bagel and lox for your lunch at my bud Mo's on sixty-ninth," the cabbie yells as I fumble with coins and folding money on the curbside.

Inside is like airport security, complete with briefcase inspection and lengthy application for a visitor's badge. As I clip it to my suit lapel, I gaze up at a hundred-plus doctors' names and room numbers confronting me. I at last locate Dr. Fereshte Ghavimi, my first port of call. There is a specialist here for each childhood cancer, assigned to do nothing but solve its particular mysteries. I will be meeting leukemia, lymphoma, neuroblastoma, and kidney specialists, a childrens' neurosurgeon, and a pathologist working solely on the genetics of childhood sarcomas.

Dr. Ghavimi is the local expert on rhabdomyosarcoma, a rare cancer which affects different muscles and responds to several newer cancer drugs. What questions can I possibly pose to her? But I needn't have worried. She proves to be a shy Iranian in an immaculately pressed white coat, who spends our first ten minutes brewing a pot of delicious tea. She smiles courteously as she offers me a tiny pot of honey.

"I assure you, doctor, this will bring out the tea's true essence."

She opens a drawer in her desk and hands me a flimsy aerogram, plus letter opener engraved with cuneiform script. The letter bears my name, c/o Sloan Kettering Cancer Center, an English stamp, and a London postmark. I ease open this mysterious envelope, and gasp at its contents.

J.S. Malpas, M.D., F.R.C.P.,
Director, Dept of Medical Oncology,
St Bartholomew's Hospital,

London, E.C.1

July 28th, 1976

Dear John,

I hope this letter finds you well, and that you are enjoying your tour of the US's major pediatric cancer centers.

My reason for seeking you out in America is to invite you to consider a consultant position in our Department of Medical Oncology at Barts. Your specific role would be to build and develop our new pediatric oncology program, which will have an inpatient unit on Kenton ward, as well as outpatient facilities to serve the greater London area. We envision your overseeing not only the clinical, but also the research and teaching aspects of this new unit.

Our sincere hope is you will consider making your formal application as soon as convenient. If you do so decide, we hope you can join us by the end of the year. Meanwhile, perhaps you could forward me your up-to-date C.V.?

Please feel free to contact me here at Barts to discuss this possibility further. You'll find my direct telephone number attached to this letter. And give my warm regards to my old friend, Don Pinkel at St. Jude's.

Yours sincerely,

J.S. Malpas, M.D., F.R.C.P.,
Director, Dept of Medical Oncology

I reread the letter three times as my astonishment expands. I am barely aware I am sitting with one of Sloan Kettering's newly minted child oncologists, who just made me a cup of unidentifiable but delicious tea. I sip absentmindedly at the brew, bringing me back abruptly to Dr. Ghavimi, who is smiling uncertainly.

"I'm terribly sorry, doctor. I . . . I . . . um . . . I've just been offered a consultant post out of the blue—a faculty attending position, you would call it. Back at my old alma mater in London, where I got my training. It's a very prestigious place." I'm almost panting, hardly able to keep my seat in front of this demure Middle Eastern lady. Back in my hotel room, I would be jumping up and down and chasing myself all round the room. "And the director himself has taken the trouble to track me down in America to make this offer. I have no idea how he knows me, or anything about me. Oh, my goodness!"

Dr. Ghavimi's smile has broadened. This whole scene has to be a first for her, too.

Boston, Philadelphia, Memphis, Houston, pass in a whirlwind. I climb in and out of planes and taxis, sign in and out at reception desks, locate offices and conference rooms, greet eminent professors with names familiar from prestigious journal articles, pursuing them through mobbed and colorful clinics and children's wards. The excitement infects me even as it transforms into familiarity. I even entertain how I might fit in here—an upstart Limey doc with a new take on the way things run in these prestigious halls of research. Where the frontiers of the war against devastating and inexplicable illnesses seem to be pushed back on a daily basis.

At each august center of excellence, the days start with resident rounds that the whole faculty attends. Not just oncologists but surgeons and pathologists, as well as invited faculty with particular expertise. The professors occupy the front benches, while the residents and students, bleary with sleep after another hectic night on call, present the case for discussion. The students wear short white coats, buttons done up for the occasion, while the residents are in operating- room scrub suits, stethoscopes stretched across their shoulders like badges of honor.

There are "visiting firemen" from other universities, too, who are treated with the same deference I quickly come to expect, however little deserved. Many feel the need to voice their opinions about the case under discussion, and what they would do differently back at "their shop." Contests break out between the faculty with the largest egos. I breathe constant sighs of relief that nobody calls on me for my opinion. After I hear "visiting firemen" a couple of times, I ask my neighbor to interpret.

"Kinda visiting hotshot," he drawls. "Some guy from outta town with a bunch of slides. Nuttin' to do with puttin' out fires. Turns out some of our native tribes have this sacred cow about another band's bigwig coming on their rez to light their fires for them. Ain't that crazy?"

I resist quizzing him about "rez"—enough ignorance betrayed for one day. Anyway, he is off at the double to yet another conference, and it is all I can do to catch up.

Time to make phone calls. My mind has been churning over the opportunities offered to me back in my homeland. The real possibility of a consultant post at Yorkhill, set against the apparent reality of one back at Barts, where the very familiarity will be more daunting than the alien culture of the West of Scotland. Let alone the dizzying diversity of America, which feels like several countries stitched together into one. Installed in Dr. Audrey Evans' office at the Childrens Hospital of Philadelphia, I hand Professor Hutchison's telephone number to her secretary. Dr. Evans, the grand lady of child cancer research, is due to meet with me at eight-thirty. It's eight in the morning here on America's east coast, so one o'clock in Glasgow. With any luck, I'll catch the prof between morning ward rounds and clinic, munching on the daily cheese-and-pickle sandwich his wife prepares for him.

"I need to reverse the charges," I tell her.

She looks at me blankly. "I mean, I wouldn't want Dr. Evans' footing the bill for me ringing up my professor in Scotland."

Her face clears. "You mean, make it collect?"

"Ah, yes, that's it. I couldn't remember the expression."

This isn't the first time I have run into weird differences between our so-called common languages. *Attorneys, apartments, trailers, trunks, hoods, trucks* . . . It might be easier if I had gone to Paris to see how things are done abroad.

"I'll 'ring him up' for you right now, doctor." The secretary grins as she dials the number. "Say, you Brits slay me with your funny expressions." She hands me the phone as soon as the call is picked up.

"Good afternoon. This is Aileen, Professor Hutchison's secretary, speaking." The educated West of Scotland accent wafting from the earpiece sounds utterly unfamiliar.

"Hallo, Aileen. John Graham-Pole speaking. How's everything?"

"Och, we're all fine. Missing you back in the old place. So how is America—pretty exciting, I'm thinking?"

"Oh, yes, wonderful. I'll tell you all about it. But . . . er . . . I wonder if Hutch is in his office?"

"I'll see if he's free."

A long moment, the phone hanging silent in my hand. I had spent a good part of the night wrestling with this complex business, and am no clearer what to hope for. My short time in America has already thrilled me with possibilities, and I have even conjured up a move across the Atlantic. But now I have this out-of-the-blue offer from Barts. It ought to feel too good to be true, but images keep flashing across my mind of my internship, and the countless humilies I experienced at the bottom of the totem pole. Could I really hold my head up as a consultant there at the tender age of thirty-four? Last, but by no means least, what if Hutch comes up with the funds to keep me on? After all, he *is* footing the bill for me to gad about the United States. If he makes me a straight offer, things will get tricky.

Hutch's gravelly voice comes on the phone. "Good afternoon, sir. Something has just come up I feel I need to let you know." I deliberately slow my words, striving to frame the situation clearly. "There was a letter waiting for me in New York, offering me a consultant position back at Barts. My medical school," I add, in case he hasn't made the link.

A long pause. "I see. And you want to take them up on their offer?"

My turn to hesitate. "It's certainly a very good one. And quite unexpected." I feel the need to scotch any suspicion I have been plotting this whole thing on this very trip he is underwriting. He relieves me of raising this particularly thorny issue.

"Well, I've looked into things, and it's not possible to create a position for you here. Regrettable, but these things must be accepted."

His terseness leaves me no room to speculate just how much regret he really feels. He has certainly been supportive, and praised me for getting published more than once, but his uneasy relationship with Willoughby speaks volumes about his skepticism towards cancer research, national treatment protocols, and the latter's latest innovation—laminar flow beds—which keep their occupants in a totally bacteria-free environment. What he would make of Arnie Freeman and the Sloan Kettering pioneers is beyond imagining.

"Well, you had better tell them you'll take it."

The conversation seems at an end. He makes no inquiries about my current activities, but has the good grace not to ask how my budget is holding up. Next morning, I catch Dr. Malpas in his Barts office. His secretary greets me like an old friend.

"He's been expecting your call. He'll be delighted to have the chance to chat."

A cultured English voice comes on the line. "John, how nice to hear from you. I was hoping you'd ring."

"I just got your aerogram when I reached New York. This is the first opportunity I've had."

"I hope you've had time to consider our offer. I've been following your career with interest since you left the old place. You've done awfully well for yourself!"

I can conjure up only a shadowy image of this man. I know he was personal assistant to Sir Ronald Bodley-Scott when I was an intern, and I would sometimes see him in the hospital square awaiting the weekly arrival of the great man's chauffeured Daimler. But how can Dr. Malpas, distinguished enough in his own right, possibly remember little old me?

"Well, I'm rather astonished—and of course delighted. I hadn't been aware there were full-time positions in pediatric oncology anywhere in Britain."

"You know, John, we rather hope we'll be first past the post. There are rumors G.O.S. may quickly follow suit."

I had been keeping in touch with friends from G.O.S. in case of such an announcement, although the idea of going back there as a consultant would be almost as daunting as a return to Barts.

Dr. Malpas continues smoothly, "There'll be the formalities, of course. An interview with some other consultants and so forth. But I don't anticipate difficulties."

No mention of salary, and it seems indelicate to raise such trivial matters. Four weeks later, I meet my would-be boss for lunch before the interview, set for two o'clock in the Dean's conference room. His continuing reassurances over further phone calls have done little to calm my jitters.

"It's such a pleasure to see you again. It's been—what, ten years? I must hear all about your grand tour. Do call me Jim, by the way."

A bowl of soup and salad is all I have appetite for, thankful not to be quizzed about my choice of dressing. The conference room proves all I've been dreading. Jim ushers me in and indicates the empty seat at the far end of the long, dark oak table. Distinguished looking men, several familiar from student days, occupy leather-seated chairs on either side. I confront the steady gaze of the dean of the medical college. He hasn't aged a day since I sat through his arduous microbiology seminars: wiry pepper-and-salt hair, horn-rimmed specs, square shoulders accentuating his height. I am acutely aware of my raw med student persona buried not too deep within my viscera.

"Good afternoon, Doctor . . ." He pauses to glance down at his notes, no doubt to get my name right. "The committee would like to pose a few questions to you. Perhaps I may start by asking your view, as an oncologist, of the Papanicolaou test for screening for cervical carcinoma."

I try to gather my wits, knowing I am at sea without a paddle. Rank unfairness: when did a child ever contract cervical cancer? And am I supposed to address him as "sir"? I hazard an answer.

"Er, I don't think its value has yet been proven, sir."

"Oh, I think you'll find its efficacy to be well proven. In fact, its use is becoming common practice."

I absorb this sniff of censure as the dean looks down the assembled ranks over his half-frame glasses. "Gentlemen, perhaps you have questions to pose to our candidate?"

After a pause, Jim comes to my rescue. "John, perhaps you might fill our committee in on your plans for pediatric oncology at Barts. Were you to be appointed, of course," he adds, in an apparent afterthought. I feel my body relax for the first time since I'd entered the room. I want to get up and shake his hand.

"I've thought about this a good deal. And of course I'm delighted that Barts has seen the value of appointing a full-time pediatric oncologist." A slight flicker of attention around the room, as if each man is taking credit for such foresight. "A dedicated ward is, I believe, essential, and you've already gone a long way towards establishing this on Kenton. The same of course goes for Outpatients. This would allow both junior doctors and nurses to get the special training needed, and to care optimally for these children."

Jim is busy nodding his head in agreement, but if anyone else around the table has any reaction, it has escaped me. I press on.

"Most important, I believe every child with cancer—suspected or proven—in the greater London area should be referred to special centers, at least for their initial work-up and treatment. It would be my job to visit all the pediatricians in the home counties to bring them up-to-date with recent advances in our field."

I sense restlessness around the room. Have I overdone it? Perhaps there is something unbecoming about stepping foot outside these hallowed walls to drum up business in said home counties. Time to pause for reactions. One of the two pediatricians—I never knew his name, let alone ever showed up for his ward rounds—breaks the silence.

"That's a very interesting concept, doctor. Do you think we have space to accommodate all these referrals you anticipate—and still leave room for children with non-fatal diseases?"

I sense I am dipping my feet into muddy waters. How do I know what the powers-that-be are planning for their pediatric department?

"I take your point absolutely. I would certainly see it as vital to discuss this with you in detail."

The dean intervenes, the handle of his specs directed down the long table toward me. Is he sensing an unseemly spat breaking out between us baby doctors?

"Perhaps you have questions you wish to pose to the committee?"

My mind blanks. What can I possibly come up with that sounds halfway intelligent? How much will they be paying me?

"I, um, I wonder about opportunities for teaching?" I stammer. "Medical students, I mean?"

It is as if I have lit a match under dry tinder. The room comes alive. I can't make out anything that anyone is saying. Heads quickly turn to other heads, everybody ignoring me. The dean makes his voice heard above the hubbub.

"Doctor, you have—quite inadvertently, I am sure—touched on a vexing issue. We are about to discuss major changes to our student teaching curriculum. There are," he pauses to lend weight, glancing about to command attention, "strongly held views on this subject. This seems a good moment to adjourn. Thank you all for sparing your precious time for this important business."

After the interview, I join Jim for a cup of tea in his office.

"Well done, John," he assures me, "I don't think there'll be any problem with your appointment."

"I hope not. I felt I stirred up something in there—about the teaching issue. What was that all about?"

"A bit of a hornet's nest, though of course you had no way of knowing. There are two camps—the more progressive consultants think we should be integrating several aspects of the curriculum—basic sciences and clinical medicine. I'm sure you remember when you crossed over from the medical college to the wards, it seemed like a journey of a thousand miles. And that nothing you had learned had any relevance to practicing medicine. The more conservative ones, though—our dean is very much in that camp—resist the kind of sweeping changes being discussed. The idea of a first-year student straight from school spending time at the bedsides to get early clinical exposure is an absolute no-no to them."

"It sounds like a pretty good notion."

"I couldn't agree more. But the problem is the students are already spread so thin, with more and more to learn every day. So having them doing a special clerkship on Kenton, let's say, learning about children with cancer, would be a challenging concept for most of those around that table. So don't hold your breath about seeing too much of our current med students."

Eight years since I fled the old place at the end of my eighteen months internship. I am still astonished to be back. Here I am at thirty-four, once more getting the hospital tour on my first day as a Barts consultant, with the dean as our tour guide: a vivid reminder of my first day on the wards as a lowly med student. He glances at me as though he has never clapped eyes on me before. There is one other new chap, who exudes confidence that will surely secure him a lucrative Harley Street private practice inside a decade.

We climb the worn stone steps of the North Wing's grand staircase—the Hogarth Stair—towards the Great Hall, as the dean recounts the story of Rahere and the Black Death, doubtless a favored topic. I take in the vastness of the hall, set off by its sparse furnishings. Polished oak table with matching chairs and a Steinway grand in one corner are the sum total. The echoes of music, coupled with visual artistry, evoke some latter-day Asclepian healing temple. My eyes rise to the scrolls gracing the Great Hall's walls: twenty generations of august benefactors, each donation recorded in precise pounds, shillings and pence. True to form, the dean trots out the time-honored dictum: "You can always tell a Barts man, but you can't tell him much."

At my first faculty meeting, I am conscious of my new wool pinstripe suit and Barts alumnus tie as I slip into an inconspicuous seat at the back. Heads swivel as the dean introduces me. I rise tentatively, unsure what is expected, but he moves swiftly to another new faculty member. Something about the broad frame of the man in the front row is familiar. As he turns to grin at the assembled company, I find myself gazing in astonishment at my ex-classmate, Jerry Gilmore, whom I haven't seen since we graduated from med school together. I have a vivid flash of heavy drinking bouts in the student bar after a hospital cup rugby game, Jerry's raucous laughter raised above everyone else's. His pleas for help before every exam, accompanied by protests that his mates had dragged him to the pub every night as he tried to hit the books. How on earth did he make it here?

But it is abundantly clear Jerry feels totally at home in this august company. As we shuffle out an hour later, I catch sight of him grasping hands and clapping backs as to the manner born. Will I ever muster such self-assurance? Do I want to?

I know after my first ward round that Sister Kenton will be laying obstacles in my path at every opportunity: a path previously untrammeled by cancer doctor upstarts. Yorkhill's nurses had always been friendly, often amused by my sassenach speech and ways, but never questioning of my decisions. If I hoped the days of nursing Sisters holding total sway in the Barts wards had become the province of the medical historians, I was about to be disillusioned. Nothing could be further from the truth—the residents and students turn out to be as cowed by Sister Kenton—"the dragon lady"—as in my day. She greets me formally at the entrance to Kenton ward, all five feet of her, arms folded tight across her bosom. Her dress is identical to that of the traditional nuns' dresses from which it derives: starched white headpiece, stiff white collar and cuffs, and the dark blue dress itself reaching to well below mid-calf. She makes no attempt to shake hands.

I am well aware of her dedication to children with advanced cancer: a dedication that takes the form of day-and-night bedside vigils, from which junior nurses and, much of the time, parents seem to be excluded. Family visiting hours are confined to one afternoon a week, relaxed only when a child is unlikely to last another twenty-four hours. This die-hard tradition must date back to medieval times at the Royal & Ancient, although why it survives baffles me. Jim Malpas has tactfully informed me that his attempts to introduce even standard chemotherapy protocols have met with Sister Kenyon's stiff resistance. He must see me as tough enough to weather the brunt of the storm—an image I am hard-pressed to picture.

The storm breaks early in my second week when I get a referral from Chris Newman in Reading. We were fellow house officers at G.O.S., then registrars together in Glasgow. He has recently been appointed as consultant pediatrician at the Royal Berks, knows about my new appointment, and has promised to send me his more challenging cases. I am delighted to hear his familiar voice on the phone.

"How are you settling in, John?"

"Well, I never thought I'd find my way back to London. It will take a while to adjust."

"I hope you'll get out here for a visit. Give us the latest cancer scoop."

"You're very much on my list. I plan on visiting all the hospitals in the home counties."

"Meanwhile, can you take a patient of mine? Four-year-old girl I admitted last night. Acute myeloblastic leukemia, white count 100,000-plus. I'm thinking of that protocol you and Mike Willoughby developed at Yorkhill. She would be a great candidate."

I make sure our isolation room is free, ask the residents to beep me as soon as the little girl, Jennifer, arrives, and meet her and her parents early that afternoon. Sister K. must have decided she is too big for a cot, so she occupies an adult-sized bed, her anxious face and blond curls scarcely visible over the neatly turned-down sheet. She makes no sound as I try to set her at ease, examining her as gently as I can. I sit on the bed's edge to talk to Mom and Dad, confirming what Chris has already told them about their daughter's diagnosis, and describing the treatment I am planning. I am acutely aware of Sister K. hovering behind my shoulder. Something in the sharp intakes of breath, the long pauses before exhalation, tells me I am in for a battle. And not just with Jennifer's leukemia.

"This treatment is going to be very hard for Jennifer—and for you both. I am very sorry to say her leukemia is the kind that is hardest to treat. And the drugs we will need to give her—the chemotherapy—are very strong. It will mean her blood counts will stay very low for many weeks, which in turn will make her prone to serious infections—in her blood and her lungs, especially. We'll need to keep her in this isolation room throughout, well away from other children."

I have learned the hard way the wisdom of not giving parents too much information at first. It has to be well-nigh impossible to make sense of anything, when you have just found out your four-year-old has an illness that may well kill her. I also know that any hope I can offer is crucial, otherwise why put anyone through what Jennifer is about to endure?

"I want to assure you, though, that I've treated quite a number of children with Jennifer's kind of leukemia, who have done very, very well. Hard to believe, perhaps, but children are in many ways tougher than us grown-ups. Their young bodies handle the kinds of chemotherapy that you and I probably couldn't." I pause to make sure this is sinking in. "The other thing I want you to be sure of: you are in no way responsible for what's happened. We don't yet know why these terrible things happen to lovely young children like your daughter. But it is absolutely nothing you did, or didn't do, that brought this on."

We are barely out of the room before Sister K. launches her attack.

"Dr. Graham-Pole, you are giving these poor parents quite unjustified hope. No one is ever cured of A.M.L. Certainly not the little ones it has been my sacred duty to nurse through their last moments. You are simply condemning her, and her parents, to needless suffering. And I've seen the effects of the treatment you propose. I cannot prevent you from conducting these kinds of *experiments*—she almost spits out the word—but I wish to register my strongest objections to your whole plan."

The residents and registrar have arrived for rounds, along with the staff nurse. No doubt they are wondering if they should make themselves scarce until the storm passes, while being covertly delighted at this showdown between the venerable old stager of our nursing profession and an untempered newcomer to the Barts consultant ranks. I struggle to cool my rising irritation and resort to reason.

"Sister, my colleagues and I recently reported on fifteen children whom we treated for A.M.L. in Glasgow. I am glad to say that fourteen of them responded, and ten of them are alive up to five years later. Yes, the chemotherapy is extreme, but anything short of this would simply postpone the inevitable."

At this moment, Jim appears at the end of the corridor. He has taken to joining us on rounds whenever he can get away, aware no doubt that occasional reinforcements will be welcome. Sister K. at once appeals to him.

"Dr. Malpas, I cannot believe what Dr. Graham-Pole is proposing for this poor little girl. I have registered my strong objection to his plan."

I already know Jim for a skilled diplomat in tricky situations. "Sister, perhaps you might rustle up a cup of tea for John and myself?"

She busies herself preparing our tea in the kitchenette off her office. She seems in no hurry, perhaps intending us to sweat it out a little. Jim and I perch on the two upright chairs by her window attempting small talk. This is the first time I have been in her inner sanctum. How much time does she spend here? For all I know, this is where she lives. She finally emerges with a teapot, three cups and saucers, and a plate of three digestive biscuits on a tray. She places everything on the oval table in the centre of the room.

"Shall I be mother? Milk, Dr. Graham-Pole?"

"Thank you, Sister."

We sip for long moments in silence. Then she launches in.

"Dr. Malpas, Dr. Graham-Pole has acquainted me with his plan of treatment for our new little patient—a patient who, I will add, has mere weeks, even days, to live. It is treatment which I consider to be highly experimental—and quite beyond anything I and my nurses have any familiarity with. I am fully aware that the final decision rests with the doctors and the parents. I am also aware that it would be unethical of me to try to sway these poor young people against your treatment plan. If I must stand aside from a decision to which I fervently object, that I will do. But I would ask you to confer with Dr. Graham-Pole, and to bring your greater experience—and, dare I say, wisdom—to bear."

Jim pauses a long moment before answering, then carefully lays his tea cup back on its saucer. "Sister, I very much respect your feelings. And of course your own immeasurable experience and compassion." Another lengthy pause, then, "However, I am personally responsible for hiring John. I did so because I knew he was breaking new ground in treating children with cancer of many kinds. I am particularly acquainted with the considerable success he has had with children with A.M.L. using combination chemotherapy. It is, of course, far from without risk, but I believe he is fully justified in choosing this course. I know you will put your personal opinions aside and give every support to our medical staff."

I might not have been in the room. The two of them regard each other in silence for a long moment. Then she lays down her own teacup.

"Very well, Dr. Malpas. I shall say no more."

"Thank you, Sister. I know this isn't easy—for any of us. And thank you for a most refreshing cup of tea."

No one had touched the digestive biscuits. I follow him out, weak with relief. Jim had backed me one hundred percent—not exactly the iron fist in the velvet glove, but close to it. Will I ever develop his skills in diplomacy? A month later, I leave the ward after morning rounds breathing lungfuls of relief. Jennifer's temperature is down for the first time in two weeks, and she is sitting up in bed with her dolls propped on pillows either side. Some God-given dispensation has allowed her to come through two rounds of my chemo protocol with only fever, sores in her mouth, and loss of every blond curl. But all the signs are that her leukemia is responding completely. Sister K. had offered not one word to the houseman's recitation of the little girl's progress. Later that afternoon, Jim proposes a pint in the Hand & Shears pub, and quickly quizzes me.

"Have you gone over with Jennifer's parents what they can expect?"

"I told them she would need three more chemo courses. And that her body should tolerate them better, now that she's in remission. I was cautiously optimistic about things, simply saying that it might never come back. But certainly no promises."

Another consultant shows up from time to time, a medical oncologist who displays especial interest in the ultra-rare forms of leukemia sometimes affecting teenagers and younger children. Jim tells me he spends a good bit of his time in the hospital's hematology laboratory, and the technicians are in the habit of quizzing him about unusual blood smears. They know to get expert input on unusual appearances down the microscope.

He is younger than most consultants, and lives up the street from where Ruth and I have just bought a house in Muswell Hill in northeast London. I get his address from the phone book, and spot his place on my way to work one morning. It is much more splendid than our own semi-detached: a three-story Edwardian surrounded by what looks like a good acre of garden, with a brand-new Jaguar XJ-12 parked in front of the double garage. The reason he can afford this life of ease becomes clear when he asks me to consult on a case of his.

"Eleven-year-old. End-stage, I'm afraid. Saudi—like a good number of my patients. And like most of them, they've left it far too late."

"Is he in Dalziel?"

I don't recall caring for any Arab patients there when I was Hamilton-Fairley's intern, but things change a lot in ten years, and I had heard of the steady flow of rich foreigners finding their way to London for second opinions among its elite cadre of medical specialists.

"Oh, no—Harley Street. London Clinic. That's where I see the bulk of my practice."

Vaguely familiar, but I have never been anywhere near Harley Street. "Medical London" has been celebrated since Victorian days for its plethora of physicians of every kind, all building lucrative practices from the huge fees they charge their wealthy clientele. I had no idea children with cancer were finding their way there.

"I'm driving over this afternoon," my colleague continues. "Perhaps we might go together. I want to be sure to cover all angles, and your particular qualifications will undoubtedly impress the family. Shall we say two o'clock in the Square?"

These last words have a hollow ring. This man has no reason to know anything about me, or my work, except that I am a pediatrician by training with some expertise in oncology. We have never even been properly introduced, and I'm not sure about the protocol for addressing him. Should I use his first name—or invite him to use mine? Far from feeling flattered, I am daunted by the prospect of treading the illustrious wards of the London Clinic. How many more well-off children and their families are finding their way to him? We drive through the streets of the City of Westminster—that ritzy section of London which I have rarely frequented—my colleague keeping up a flow of gossip about goings-on among the Barts consultant staff, most only names to me.

"I'm planning a move closer to town, now my private practice is taking off so well. People are finding their way to us from all over the map."

I am grateful he doesn't quiz me on my own intentions. On my salary as the most junior consultant, I am all too aware of the size of my mortgage. He parks the Jag outside an elegant Georgian building, with bowers of flowers bedecking its balconies, and a Union Jack fluttering in the breeze above.

"Welcome to The Clinic, doctor."

It turns out to be more like a hospital than the usual Harley Street consulting rooms—but unlike any I have ever seen—more my idea of a smart West End hotel. A sophisticated receptionist greets us in the hallway, a porter slides open the elevator doors, and we are swept upwards to the third floor where the children's ward is located.

"Good afternoon, Sister. This is my colleague, Dr. Graham-Pole. I've asked him to consult on my newest admission."

Sister offers me a deferential smile, something I have yet to encounter among Barts senior nursing staff, as she ushers us into a room at the end of the ward. There are several people gathered in the small space. A man in traditional Arab white tunic and headdress bows in silent greeting as we enter. Behind him, I count three women in full-length black dresses, all veiled so that only their eyes are visible through narrow slits. In the subdued light, I eye a child huddled on the bed under what looks like a cross between an eiderdown and a rich Persian rug. As I approach him, I spot beads of sweat on his scalp. Then I take in another figure curled up on the floor beneath the bed—a man of sub-Saharan origin from what I can take in.

"The boy's slave," my colleague murmurs.

Does he really mean that—*his slave*?

My brief exam tells me the boy is not long for this world. He is emaciated, feverish, and covered in bruises the length and breadth of his body. Both his liver and spleen are huge and craggy, stretching from under his diaphragm down into his distended belly. He stays silent throughout my exam, apart from a soft moaning as I palpate his abdomen. As I straighten up, Sister proffers his temperature chart. He has been here five days, and his fever has been raging between 102° and 104° ever since admission. I read off the cocktail of potent antibiotics he has been receiving around the clock. Catching the inscrutable collective gaze of the several family members, I am at once clear I won't be able to carry on a conversation with any of them. Anyway, what on earth would I say to these people who have travelled all the way from Saudi Arabia on such a futile quest?

"Perhaps you would wish to review his blood samples, Dr. Graham-Pole," Sister offers. "Our laboratory is at the end of the hallway. I will convey your opinion to our interpreter, who will be joining us shortly."

I glance again at the family, who are talking among themselves in a rising murmur, as I follow my colleague through the door Sister is holding open. I gaze down the microscope at the clusters of malignant white corpuscles crowding the blood smear, almost displacing anything resembling a healthy cell.

"White count 210,000 this morning," my colleague offers. "I'm no pediatrician, but I make that about twenty times the normal number for an eleven-year-old. From what I can gather from his reports, he's had about nine months of chemotherapy. And already relapsed twice after what sound like transient remissions. It's doubtful he ever responded completely." He glances up from his notes. "I take it you haven't any other tricks up your sleeve?"

"I'm very much afraid it would be an exercise in futility. He looks as if he could die at any moment. Any more hefty chemotherapy would undoubtedly kill him—long before it had any chance of altering the course of his leukemia."

"I already told them that. But I've also assured them you are one of the nation's leading childhood leukemia specialists—and that the buck stops with you. I'm not sure how the interpreter translated that," he adds as an afterthought. "Well, they want to try to get him home before it's too late. I think they have a private jet waiting. Do you think you could get a cab back to Barts? I've a few more patients to see. The receptionist will whistle one up for you."

He shakes my hand before thrusting a thick sealed envelope towards me. "Many thanks for all your help, doctor. I'm sure I'll be calling on you again."

I open the envelope in the taxi. It holds six crisp new £50 banknotes. All that for an unnecessary ten-minute consultation. It feels like tainted money.

Chapter 6: *VENTURING*

I start making regular trips back to G.O.S., my old haunt. Jon Prichard is fresh from a year's fellowship at Dana Farber in Boston and has just been appointed as a full-time oncologist there. So now there are two of us in the country, and the scene looks set for dialogue and cooperation, assuming territorial rivalries don't get in our way. Having served time in the training ranks of both places—Barts and G.O.S.—I know politics can readily raise its ugly head. Easy to envision what kind of competitive instincts may emerge when two brand new pediatric oncology units open up within a mile of each other. Statistics tell us that one in ten thousand children will develop any kind of cancer, so a pretty small number will fall victim in all six home counties on any given Tuesday.

Jon welcomes me warmly. He has established weekly teaching rounds for the whole staff, but he is hoping to attract interested outsiders. There is an obvious American flavor to the set-up, and I find myself fitting in comfortably. It is a welcome relief from the very British style of our Barts conferences. These are focused entirely on adult cancers, and all they do for me is evoke grim memories of my intern year with Gordon and Neville.

I get to present Jennifer, my four-year-old patient with A.M.L., and talk about our success treating these children in Glasgow. John tells me about a plan to start a children's oncology group in Britain. John Martin, the senior pediatrician at Alder Hey Children's Hospital in Liverpool, and Pat Morris-Jones at Manchester Children's Hospital, have organized a day to explore pooling our efforts. They have both been giving chemo to children with solid cancers—kidney and bone and brain tumors—to supplement the surgery and radiotherapy that were until recently standard treatment. Several of us have had spells in the United States, and all agree that it is high time we caught up with our American colleagues.

Towards the end of the year, Jon and I join our colleagues in Liverpool. The day ends with a pub meal washed down with pints of local beer, and we barely make it to Lime Street station in time for the nine-thirty back to Euston. We head to the bar to talk about our day. We are soon comparing notes about our own programs back in London, and after a second Whitbread's Pale we are both loosening up. The competition for the same pool of patients remains an unspoken constraint, but both of us at Barts and G.O.S. have our own followings, which may prove an amicable solution. Most children with leukemia are being referred to G.O.S., which is much more familiar to the area's pediatricians. But we are getting a steady referral of teenagers, among whom lymphomas and sarcomas—cancers of bone and muscle—are commoner, the medical oncologists being quick to send them on to us. I quiz Jon about his year in America, and whether he would ever want to work there permanently.

"It's certainly exciting in the States. Hard to get the same buzz going back here in London. But this new job is keeping me busy—and things are growing fast. What about you?"

"Well, I'm keeping in touch with friends I made over there. And parts of the London scene bother me quite a bit. I was shocked to find children from the Middle East showing up in the London Clinic—referred to adult oncologists, I may say. The families end up paying oodles of money under the table, only to be told their child's cancer is way too advanced for treatment, and they had best take an early plane home, lest their child die on foreign soil."

"Wow, I had no idea. You certainly don't see anything like that in America. The medical oncologists have all the work they need, without trying to take on stuff that's out of their league. So what about you? You ever considered a move across the pond?"

"Well, I had a great time there. I'm pretty isolated at Barts, to be honest. Adult oncology is definitely not my thing—I found that out during internship. And it's an uphill battle with our nursing staff. They are pretty set in their ways, and very far from supporting me in trying new treatment approaches. We'll see how things work out."

At the end of my first Barts year, Sister K. announces her intention to retire.

"I'm too old to change, Dr. Graham-Pole. These new treatments you are using, well, I'll never accept them. They cause the children far too much pain and distress, and to what end? How many will survive?"

"I know we have had our differences, Sister. And you're absolutely right, the children do suffer a great deal—as do their families." I hesitate, wondering if we can perhaps find some common ground. "But there are more and more treatments being developed, and we are getting many of the children back to living close to normal lives. At least for a time."

She shakes her head. "Perhaps we must agree to differ, Dr. Graham-Pole."

Jim tells me about the party he is planning at his home to say goodbye to Sister K. After thirty years of selfless service, her reputation is far-reaching, and he expects a full complement of senior nurses to show up, as well as many consultants. When I arrive, I am surprised to find her polishing off a large glass of sherry and looking about for a refill. The very first time I've seen her out of her Sister's uniform: she is wearing a modest short-sleeved grey dress that hangs just below her knee. She greets me with more warmth than I ever remember encountering.

"Dr. Graham-Pole, I'm happy to see you here. I thought perhaps, with our occasional differences of opinion, you might decide to give my party a miss."

"I wouldn't have missed it for the world, Jackie." This is the first time I have taken the liberty of addressing her by her first name. I quickly regret the tenor of my response—as though I am overjoyed to be present at her departure. But I am reassured by the twinkle in her eye.

"I shall be retiring to my country home in Mousehole. Cornwall, you know, right on the coast. Perhaps you'll come visit, bring me up to date with your latest experiments."

"I'd be delighted to take you up on your kind invitation."

Very much a changing of the guard. I have already met her replacement, a woman in her late thirties. This will be her first post as a ward sister, and she seems open to the ideas I have tentatively mentioned to her. I talk with Jim about attending the big gathering of American oncologists the following April.

"John, I think our success with treating children with Ewing's and other sarcomas would make a very nice paper for Washington. They have a separate section for childhood cancers—and we can both catch up with old friends."

Once I have submitted my proposal to give a paper, I spend my spare time reading everything published on chemotherapy for children with sarcomas, preparing charts and graphs to display our results. Early January, the letter arrives to say I've been accepted for a special session entitled "Solid Pediatric Tumors." I feel a buzz of excitement as I book flights and a hotel in the nation's capital. Jim has gone ahead to visit his old friend, Don Pinkel, in Memphis, so I am on my own. The cab driver points out the sights as we drive along the Potomac from the airport. Spring is in full bloom and the cherry blossoms are stunning.

"Lincoln Memorial, sir. F.D.R., Jefferson Memorial, all our presidents are remembered. That's the Washington Monument. Our city is the most beautiful in the world."

This man is nothing like the fast-talking, fast-driving cabbies I remember from New York. But he obviously didn't start out life here.

"Where are you from, originally?"

"Ethiopia, sir. Many Ethiopians here."

"Are you a citizen, then?"

"Oh, yes, sir. My family came when I was twelve. You must visit our restaurant."

That night I stroll from the Capitol building up the National Mall, ending my walk at the White House gates, then take the metro to my cabbie's family restaurant. The food is spicy and delicious, and I wash it down with wine that tastes of honey. Looking at my map, I relish the thirty-minute stroll back to the hotel. Back in the foyer, I scan the conference details for the next day on the lit-up screens, aware of the buzz around me. I finally retire to my room, too revved up to sleep. I'm up at 5 a.m. to stroll out and watch the city awakening.

The pediatric sessions are not until the third day, and Jim Malpas and I part company after the early-morning keynotes. I am both alarmed and excited by the combative dialogue following every presentation. I am swept along with the crowds trying to squeeze into the more cutting-edge sessions. How many of them are dealing with nursing sisters out to block every new therapy developed? I hook up with a group of oncologists from Philadelphia, while Jim is off with the small Barts contingent.

"We'd sure welcome some of you Brits here," one dinner companion tells me. "Shake up our thinking, import some new ideas."

"I'd have to do my residencies again, wouldn't I?"

"Hell, no. From what you're saying, you've got more training under your belt than most of our assistant profs. What year d'you graduate?"

"1966."

"Say, that's a long time, buddy. You ever consider emigrating, give us a call. Be happy to look over your C.V."

On my way back to my hotel, I stop at a bar near Dupont Circle. Someone had mentioned *The Big Hunt* has about every beer imaginable. I take a table opposite a woman obviously on her own. A few years older than me, cropped dark hair, no make-up. There is a look of freedom about her. She starts talking at once.

"You're at the cancer convention, right?"

"How d'you know?"

"I can always spot doctors." Midwest accent, definitely not East Coast. "You an oncologist?"

"Pediatric, actually. There's a few of us. John."

"Barbara. You're a Brit?"

"From London. You?"

"Medical writer for a pharmaceutical company. Always cover these conventions. So tell me about your work, John."

I'm quickly opening up to her, spilling my life story.

"So why oncology? Pediatrics, especially?"

"Goes back to my Mom's death. When I was twelve."

The first time in my adult life I have ever openly acknowledged this to anyone. I am seized by a desperate impulse to burst into tears, but it feels once I start I won't be able to stop. Barbara senses my distress.

"Where you staying?"

"The Hilton."

"Me too. Let's get out of here."

We spend the night in her room, alternating between lovemaking and talking—and, in my case, crying my eyes out. I had no idea I had these many tears to shed. It's like I have opened a door slammed shut twenty-five years before to allow a torrent of grief to pour forth. Barbara lets it flow as I talk, and talk some more. The huge weight of thoughts and feelings crammed down deep gradually lightens. I am left with a sense of immeasurable relief. Repeat performances follow the next two nights, but laughter now replaces the tears. Barbara produces two expertly rolled joints, and at thirty-six years old I take my very first puff. We are quickly rolling about the bed in hysterics for no fathomable reason. I am filled with a joy I can never before recall. When we wake on our last morning, it is to the realization of two things: I have discovered for the first time in my life what it means to fall hopelessly in love; and I am due on the overnight flight back to London.

I cannot face Ruth in the days after my homecoming. Hard even sharing our bed. I drink heavily each evening and turn in late, then rise early to care for the children. Ruth is no morning person, so she is happy to hand over these chores. George, Kate, and I relish our uninterrupted hour or more before she makes it down for a swift breakfast before I leave for work.

I take to phoning Barbara at home in Columbus, Ohio, each day at eleven o'clock, G.M.T.—6 a.m. for her—before she heads off to her pharmaceutical job. We exchange a steady stream of life stories, Barbara telling me about her two teenagers, Julie and Amy, and how it has been to share them with her ex-husband for several years. I am filled with impatience until it is time to place the next call from the shelter of my hospital office. As soon as I hear her voice, I am back in our Washington hotel room, filled with longing for the solace of her arms about me. Just what is it in her that has wrought such a sea change in my every thought and action? And how on earth will Ruth and I ever be able to reach any kind of amicable arrangement? I spend lunchtimes at a pub opposite the Old Bailey law courts, downing pints and pouring out page after page to her, and a week after my return I am reading her own equally ardent letter back.

I somehow manage to focus my mind on my work, seeing new patients, running my clinic, handling consult requests, and talking to pediatricians at referring hospitals. A phone call comes from the head chap in the Radiotherapy Department.

"Will you see a patient of mine? I'm treating him for bone cancer—mostly for pain control. But now it's in both lungs. Thought perhaps your new protocols might have something to offer."

We meet over Brian's X-rays. I recall my colleague from intern days—he must be twice my age. I sense at once his lack of faith in chemotherapy, and by extension chemo docs. One look tells me his seventeen-year-old patient has a couple of months, tops, and that chemo would be a futile exercise. It might buy him a short spell, but at the cost of miserable side effects. I reflect on how different it might have been if I had seen Brian at the beginning of his illness, when starting an intensive chemo regimen might just have saved his life.

"Maybe I could meet the family first?"

"You want the boy there? He's a minor, has no idea what's up."

"Yes, I'd like to bring him in on this."

I sense more skepticism, but he ushers me into Brian's room on Dalziel, introduces the father, then sweeps out with his student entourage. Brian's head is turned to the window, while Mom sits close by his bed. It flashes on me: no one has ever told me how to do this. All those doctor-patient conversations, but the only time I have heard the C-word, let alone the D-word, was out of Quint's lips in Norwich. So the buck stops here. I am flying solo and will just have to wing it. I pull my chair close to Brian's bedside and offer my hand. He twists around, pain in every movement. Dread, too. His face is sallow, bereft of youthfulness. He hesitates, then shakes my hand briefly. I hold his look.

"Hi. John Graham-Pole's my name. I work with people your age. Dr. Stafford asked if I could see you. What's he told you, I wonder? About your illness?"

"Hasn't talked to me."

Clipped middle-class accent—a younger version of myself.

I glance across at Mom, then over my shoulder at Dad. Their faces are frozen. Perhaps terrified I'll break the unspoken code and bring up Brian's diagnosis?

"What about you both? What have you understood?"

Mom hesitates, then: "He said Brian needed special drug treatments, to help the X-ray therapy. Is that what you do, doctor?"

"Yes. But other things, too. I can help with Brian's pain, hopefully get him up and about again." I turn back to their son. "Are you getting enough pain meds?"

He shakes his head no.

"I can fix that. How about sleeping?"

Another shake.

"I can help there, too. Maybe work on your appetite—not too good, right?"

"Can't eat. Too sick after those treatments."

"Right. We've some stuff for that, too. When did you last get home?"

"Couple of weeks."

"Any friends been around?"

"Yeah, a couple. Once. Too far to come."
"Where d'you live?"
"Basingstoke."
Stockbroker belt. A lengthy train ride.
"Yeah, that'd be a trip."
"Anyway, they're away at college."
"So you're missing a few classes?"
"Yup." A ghost of a grin. A first.

"Brian, I'm going to order up pain medicines, help you sleep, then chat with your parents about the drugs." I hesitate. "I'll be back to talk more when you're more rested. I'll tell you all about possible treatments we can give." I pause again. "And anything else you want to know."

I sense heightened tension in the room. But Brian is holding my look, like that would be just fine with him. Like no one has told him a dicky-bird.

The almoner's room is free. His parents start to talk, hesitant at first, then freely, about what they've been told—or not. Mom does most of it, then Dad joins in, as they take turns pouring out their fears, and their anger. Mom begins, "It's always 'lump'—at most 'growth'. Now he has these 'lung and back problems'. That's it—that's all we get."

"Like we're stupid."

"Everyone avoids the word. Cancer."

I sense her surprise at letting slip the word. *Light bulb*: listening is a whole lot easier than talking. I ease my grip on my chair, hold each one's look in turn, letting them know I'm not going anywhere. The hard questions pour out in a rush.

"Do we have a choice, doctor? About this chemotherapy? What's going to happen? How will it be? What do we tell him?"

I allow a long pause before answering. "Yes, you have choices. I suggest you talk together. Don't rush. But Brian should know what's up. I think he knows already."

Panic in Mom's eyes. "We can't tell him! Can you talk to him, doctor?"

"Yes, I'll look after that. And everything else. Whatever happens."

The questioning ends. I make my way back to Brian's room, rehearsing the conversation: where I'll sit, what I'll say for openers. I am all too aware this will be the first time I have talked candidly to a teenager about his fatal illness.

But Brian makes it easy. No sooner have I perched on the chair close to his bed that he starts talking. "I know all about what's going on. What's wrong with me. About the X-rays and stuff."

"So what are you thinking?"

"That I'm not going to make it. Drugs or no drugs."

I stay quiet, sensing the futility of filling the space with reassuring words. Knowing silence itself can speak volumes.

"I'm okay, doctor," Brian says at last. "I'm just worried about my parents."

"I've been talking to them. They'll be okay, too. And they know I am talking to you about what's up. They said it's up to you—whether we try these drugs or not."

"What'll happen? Will they make me sick, like the radiation?"

"Yes, Brian, they will. We would have to give you a pretty powerful combination to have a chance of making a dent in your cancer. You'll be very nauseous, get the runs, have mouth sores, won't want to eat, lose a good bit of weight."

"Will it make much difference? To the cancer?"

"I don't know, Brian. But it's maybe worth a try. If you're up for it."

"I just don't want to go on hurting. My back's pretty bad. I can't sleep. And even my breathing feels hard."

"Yes. The cancer is in both your lungs and your spine. I'm going to give you morphine, Brian, on a regular schedule. It'll not only lift your pain, it will make breathing easier, and help take your anxiety away."

"I'm not scared, doctor. Thanks for helping me. And Mom and Dad."

I have no answer, knowing if I try I will start crying. Which is just what Brian doesn't need. We end up giving him that try, mostly I suspect because he doesn't want to let his parents down—or even me. He does indeed get very sick, and every day feels more futile. After two rounds of chemo, we repeat the X-rays: minimal if any change. By this time, Brian looks like he is at death's door, and he is refusing to eat. I feel secret relief that we won't have to persist with this charade. He dies peacefully a week after receiving his final chemo shot. His last words to me are a murmured thank you.

Six weeks since I returned from Washington. Weeks of avoiding Ruth, of daily conversations with Barbara, of putting in full days at work with a growing patient load, plus working on academic papers. I am spending every early morning and evening with George and Kate, who are growing fast and filling me with joy at acquiring new words and skills, then drinking after Ruth goes to bed, writing to Barbara, re-reading her letters to me. One Friday night, after the children are asleep, Ruth confronts me.

"I want to know what's going on, John. You've hardly opened your mouth this month. You've got plenty of time for the children, but none at all for me."

We are sitting at opposite ends of the kitchen table. I feel only relief she has forced the issue. I can't duck this any longer.

"I met someone—in America. I've been talking to her every day. I can't go on living like this. I want to move there."

Silence at first, then Ruth erupts into a spate of furious questions, not pausing for any response. How could I possibly abandon her with two young children, fly off thousands of miles? How will she cope for money? Have I not one scrap of conscience? I'm totally crazy, utterly irresponsible. The tirade rushes on. I sit silent, letting it blow over me, waiting for it to subside, every word out of her mouth adding weight to my guilt.

I can't even begin to think about my loss of George and Kate. Will she ever let me see them? Even if she does, how will I bear the greater part of my life apart from them? But through it all I know I've got to do this. Somehow find a way to cope with such a seemingly unendurable loss.

Ruth's anger explodes again when we head up to bed. I end up heading back downstairs to the sitting room sofa, unable to sleep for the churning mix of guilty, sad, yet excited feelings. Three days later, I pack a single suitcase and move in with a friend of a friend. I send off more than twenty letters to U.S. pediatric oncology centers, receive several encouraging replies. A firm offer arrives from a Dr. Sam Gross at Rainbow Babies & Childrens Hospital in Cleveland, Ohio. I find a map in the library and confirm that Cleveland is only a hundred miles north-east of Columbus. I can hardly believe my good fortune.

I book an all-expenses-paid flight and meet with Sam and his colleagues—two other women oncologists, both younger than me—before spending a joyful reunion weekend with Barbara. In Cleveland, everything goes smoothly, and I meet countless colleagues in a flurry of handshakes. Back at work, I get the confirmation letter offering me an Associate Professor position starting December, 1978, salary $35,000 annually. Equivalent to almost twice my current earnings. I meet with Jim for a drink after work in the Hand and Shears.

"Jim, I've some rather difficult news to impart. I've been exploring possibilities in the States, and—to cut to the chase—I want to accept a position in Cleveland, Ohio."

"John, I've had the feeling things haven't been entirely happy for you here. You've done excellent work, and it's great you have got several publications in good journals. Well, these things happen. You have put in two years, and it hasn't been at all easy. I shall certainly continue to follow your career with great interest, and I wish you every success. Do you have a date in mind?"

"They would like me to start in December, if that works at your end. I realize it's putting a big burden on you, but I thought two months notice seemed fair."

"Absolutely fine, John. Thanks so much for being so straightforward with your plans."

I am somewhat deflated at how easily Jim has accepted my news. But I know my recent behavior has been erratic, with my keeping long office hours and disappearing to the pub every lunch time. And he has perhaps noticed the daily trans-Atlantic calls from my office, though he has had the grace never to mention it. We part on cordial terms in late November, promising to keep in close touch.

Ruth reluctantly agrees to my spending an afternoon with George and Kate before I fly. I have no clear idea how often I'll be able to see them, how often I can get away from my new position, let alone afford the cost of transatlantic travel. Will she let them travel unaccompanied? I'll be wiring most of my monthly salary to her after keeping enough for my own immediate expenses, but I daren't think through all the huge uncertainties.

I try to explain to George why I am living in this strange flat, and why I can't come home, but it is too much for him to grasp. Especially my wanting to just hug and hug them both tight, and weep, rather than play the way we always used to. Two-year-old Kate is content to eat her tea, then fall asleep on my lap after I've read the first two pages of her new picture book. I drop them back at the house and hurry away, listening to the sound of my heart breaking.

As I wade through the sidewalk drifts between Rainbow Babies &

Children's hospital and the downtown bus stop, freezing sleet coats me to mid-calf. I have yet to purchase snow-proof boots. No word on when the car I bought in London will arrive, but I will have to pick it up on the Baltimore docks. Shivering in the shelter, I take in I'm the only white person among the dozen or so other huddlers. Every sight and sound is alien, and I abandon any attempt to follow my companions' conversations.

My mind is numb. I hardly dare contemplate my situation. My new boss had taken me on ward rounds with him on my second work day. As I tuned into the conversation in the doctors' room where the residents present the current inpatients, I could grasp only the barest outline. Histories, physicals, lab tests, plans for the day all presented at breakneck speed, giving me only a foggy notion of each ailment or treatment plan. It is not only the alien language but their fast talk and weird jargon. Almost every patient is on Tylenol, but shyness prevents my asking for translation (Panadol in England, I later discover). I have been hired as an Associate Professor, expected to teach these self-assured young men and women something they don't already know. What have I dropped myself into?

I cry myself to sleep each night. I miss George and Kate desperately, and my guilt is overwhelming. My one attempt to phone them, using my office phone, is disastrous. All I get is a tirade from Ruth about my appalling behavior, abandoning her in desperate financial straits. I tell her I will wire money with my first paycheck, omitting the horrendous difficulties of setting this up without even a social security number or U.S. driving license. She is adamant I can't talk to the children until they have started adjusting to this ghastly situation I alone have created. All this carried on amidst dread that the secretaries are listening in, eager for clues about a Limey doc trading his life in London—every American working girl's dream trip—for this "mistake on the lake," as Cleveland is freely labeled.

I keep my nightly phone conversations with Barbara short, aware I am dependent on new colleague Susan Shurin's hospitality. She refuses my attempts to offer room and board, but is clearly not expecting this to be a long term arrangement. I have arranged to take off the week between Christmas and New Year, and I spend Christmas Day at Barbara's home, meeting sixteen-year-old Julie and thirteen-year-old Amy. I do my best to put on a cheerful face, but my mind keeps spinning back to the familiarity of English festivities. Christmas without turkey—apparently reserved for Thanksgiving—nor even Brussels sprouts or roast chestnuts. Most of the time

I feel like a child of six in desperate need of Mom.

Barbara and I drink too much, which only opens distance between us. We have booked a ski vacation in West Virginia, but there is no repeat of the recent snow storms, and most of the slopes and trails prove to be closed, so our first trip together proves a dismal failure. Early on the first of January, I take the prop plane back to Cleveland, ever more fearful for the future. My next weekend in Columbus is almost a repeat of the last, and the night before I am due back at work, Barbara and I face the options. My total dependency—having her play essentially full-time therapist—is stifling her. I hadn't anticipated the extent of my culture shock and am terrified at the thought of just giving up and heading back home. Articulating my feelings in any coherent way proves nigh impossible; demons are surfacing for both of us.

I find out belatedly that she has already had three husbands, and three divorces. Could that have been an early-warning sign? Back in Cleveland, I talk to Sam about my difficulties, which he seems to grasp. He hasn't put me on call yet, and without much clinical work or research plans, I spend my days in my office poring over complex and largely alien patient treatment protocols. Susan lends me her car to explore the city, get a bank account, and find an apartment. My efforts at Barts have told me I have no bent for laboratory research, but the immunopathology director gives me space to freeze samples of fresh neuroblastoma cells. I have a notion to embark on testing new chemicals with cancer-killing properties, although I am hazy about where I will obtain them.

As I start to settle in, I attend my first Tumor Board meeting, where we discuss recent patient referrals with our pathologist, radiologist, and pediatric surgeons. I'm on familiar ground, and get the sense I am as knowledgeable as anyone about current treatment approaches to the patients being discussed. I find an affordable apartment in Shaker Heights, and get word my new M.G.B. has arrived in Baltimore. I make plans to fly down next weekend, relishing the four-hundred-mile return journey. Having my own vehicle will make a huge difference to the commute between Cleveland and Columbus. Barbara and I are exploring possibilities for her working here, or even my finding a position in Ohio State's pediatric oncology division, though so far with little encouragement on either end.

Every children's specialty is represented at Rainbow. Not just neonatology, cardiology and nephrology, but immunology and endocrinology and even pediatric orthopedics. Most requests to consult on other faculty members' patients are for hematology issues that I am poorly equipped to answer. Pediatric oncology has been my sole preoccupation for five-plus years, with hematology mostly a closed book. I ponder questions like, "What is the significance of this thirteen-year-old's low hemoglobin?" "Is it safe to operate on this infant with a mildly extended bleeding time?" "Why does this seven-year-old with rheumatoid arthritis have a persistently high white count?" I have rarely addressed any of these issues, certainly not as "the expert." I sneak peeks at my hematology colleagues' several-page reports, painfully aware that my own scribbled efforts lack any definitive recommendations.

On my first teaching rounds, I realize the residents don't know as much as their confident demeanors project. But they pick up fast how foreign their medical terminology is to me. They giggle at my cute vernacular while finding my opinions and orders mostly weird. Not just the alien terms, but their many accepted clinical practices are often at odds with my own training. I am bewildered at the speed everything moves. I catch myself standing at the nurses' station watching everyone tear off on urgent missions, shouting alien orders, and trading jokes I can't begin to follow.

Making phone calls to referring doctors' offices in unknown towns without the advantage of seeing their faces is still harder: I am acutely aware of my B.B.C. accent as I flounder through these conversations. Culture shock is a term I've only vaguely heard, but it hits me I have a bad case. My every familiar social and psychological experience and sensation, essential to day-to-day functioning, has been abruptly replaced by an alien and dissonant jangle of voices, sights, smells, sensations. The D.S.M. (*Diagnostic and Statistical Manual of Mental Disorders*), the world's authority on psychological illnesses, may not list my condition, but I know when I'm sick.

Unable to share my pent-up feelings with my colleagues, I find myself gaining solace from an unanticipated source: my patients. They have no notion I am at sea without a sail, it's a big whoopee for them to trade jokes as they test their best limey lines for my approval. I start sneaking back to sit on their beds at day's end when the ward is largely empty bar the nursing night shift and the odd intern. The parents grab the chance to take off for a smoke, while I learn new games and silly TV shows. I even talk about life in England, and my own teenage years. Tears often prick at my eyelids, but if they notice they don't seem the least troubled. It is from them that I learn about Ohio's geography, because most hail from small towns surrounding the metropolis.

As I grow more comfy with their vernacular, I venture to lift whole phrases into later dialogues with my colleagues. George Bernard Shaw may have been right that the U.S. and Britain are two countries separated by a common language, but I am picking up enough American jargon to get by.

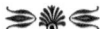

Sam and I meet with two medical oncologists, Roger and Hillard, to set up a bone marrow, or stem cell, transplant unit, primarily to treat our leukemia patients. We decide that we will offer it to both adults and children for whom more standard treatments have failed. We all know the children will tolerate better than adults the extreme treatments needed to get the transplanted stem cells to engraft in the patient, and to offer a possible cure, but Sam tells me very few U.S. children's centers have ventured into this field. Such specialized units mean major financial investment, primarily because these patients need round-the-clock nursing for six weeks and often longer while they recover from their intensive regimens of chemo and whole-body radiation. They must be nursed in laminar air flow units to keep the air surrounding them sterile, and receive non-absorbed oral antibiotics to sterilize their bowels and cut down the high risk of sepsis from bacteria penetrating bowel walls that the chemo inevitably damages.

Most pediatricians are reluctant to put their patients through this "kill or cure" approach, but Sam and I agree that, for the hardest-to-treat cancers, *more* definitely is *better*. Delivering several times the normal chemo doses, followed by infusing healthy marrow stem cells, may well cure an otherwise incurable patient. Roger already has a national reputation in this field, and is treating patients with a combination of eight different drugs at once—essentially all those known to kill leukemia cells. Patients start being referred from all over northern Ohio, and soon further afield, and Sam is happy to let me take the lead in setting up the unit for our first child patients.

What gets my attention is Roger's technique for freezing stem cells from the patients' own marrows, once they are in remission from their initial chemotherapy. He uses liquid nitrogen to freeze and preserve their stem cells at super cold temperatures (-196° centigrade), which can keep them alive until we have finished our otherwise lethal doses of chemo to kill their remaining cancer cells. This technique is called autologous (self), distinguishing it from regular allogeneic transplants, which require a well-matched sibling donor. It avoids several problems with another person's marrow: either rejection of the engrafted stem cells or so-called graft-versus-host disease, caused by the donor cells attacking the patient's skin and bowel—tissues that it sees as foreign—while the patient's immune system is severely suppressed.

My mind goes back to the children with neuroblastoma Jon Pritchard and I had treated with very high doses of a rarely used chemo drug called melphalan, and which Jon is getting ready to report on. So what if we froze marrow stem cells from similar children, once we've put them into remission? Could we not give them otherwise lethal doses of chemo plus whole-body radiation before reinfusing their stem cells, just as with our leukemia patients? I can find no evidence anywhere in the medical literature that such approach has ever been used to treat children with advanced and uniformly fatal neuroblastoma.

Meanwhile, another interest that I had developed in London—that of treating bone cancers with high chemo doses—takes a new turn. John Makely, an orthopedist I had met at our tumor conferences, asks me to join him in Radiology to see one of his patients. I read off her name, Brandy, on the X-ray film. An extensive cancer is completely replacing her right shoulder joint and extending halfway down its shaft.

"Fourteen-year-old with osteosarcoma. See where I biopsied it. And this girlie's got an additional problem. She's been deaf from birth, relies entirely on sign language to communicate. It'll be a major problem if we do the standard amputation of her whole arm to be sure to get the whole cancer. So I wonder what's your experience with limb-salvage procedures?"

"I've not done any myself, and certainly not heard of it for a proximal humeral cancer. Are you leaning that way?"

"All for it, if you're game. You've got good drugs to shrink these things, don't you?"

"Yes, they're having great results in Boston and Sloan Kettering, and in Europe too. Giving the first few doses upfront to shrink down the cancer to make your job of resecting it a whole lot easier. Neoadjuvant chemotherapy, they call it. And in Brandy's case, it could save her hand and forearm, and not interfere with her using sign language. I'd love to try. Have you talked to her family?"

"Only in outline. Thought we'd best do that together."

We meet Brandy and her parents next day. Her arm is in a sling, but Mom says it's fine to remove it so I can get a good look. I take the remaining chair and smile at Brandy as I examine her. A sheen of dread crosses her face as she glances quickly at her mother. The huge swelling of her right arm mirrors her X-rays, extending almost to her elbow. I avoid pressing on the lump, or seeing how far she can move her shoulder. Mom signs to her daughter continuously, while John stands in the window. I realize how rarely I have seen surgeons sit down.

"Mr. and Mrs. Andrews, Dr. Makely asked me to talk to you. I know he's already explained about Brandy's condition and the possible treatments."

"Yes, doctor." Her mother goes on signing to Brandy as she speaks. "He said he'd usually plan on an amputation, but you could give her your chemotherapy drugs first, so he might not have to."

"Yes, that's exactly what we're thinking about. But it's a very new treatment and we haven't had a case like your daughter's, so we can't make promises. Brandy always uses both hands for signing, right?"

"Well, she *could* perhaps learn to use one hand. But it would be very confusing for her—really like learning a new language. All her friends at the deaf school she goes to use both hands to talk. Maybe I could ask her?"

"If it won't upset her too much, I'd like to know what she thinks."

Their signed conversation goes back and forth for several long minutes. Brandy gets more and more agitated, while Mom looks ready to tear up as she turns back to me. I have got the gist.

"It'd be very hard for her, for all of us. We really want you to try the chemo first."

"Thank you, Mrs. Andrews. I'm sorry to upset you both. We can start our treatment right away, and you can stay with Brandy. There will be some papers to sign, once you're in the ward."

We give Brandy four rounds of a chemo combination I am very familiar with, but upping the doses according to our newest protocols. She seems to have no idea she is the subject of such a unique experiment. Her pain and swelling diminish quickly, and it becomes much easier for her to move her right arm. Two months after I had first met her, she can raise it to brush her hair—what is left of it. Meanwhile, I have mastered a few sign words, although I can't translate any of the sounds coming from her lips. John and I meet once more over her X-rays.

"It's worked far better that I ever expected," he announces. "You've made a convert of me. The whole thing looks dead as potato chips. I'm scheduling her for surgery next week, okay?"

"Absolutely. Her blood counts are back up after the last chemo course, and everything else is functioning fine. You think you'll be able to save her hand?"

"You bet. Everything suggests I can resect any remaining cancer, then get good bony and soft tissue union. We've got these new microvascular techniques, and the latest titanium implants look real good. Sure be fascinating to see how much tumor necrosis we find."

Three days after surgery, Brandy is once more happily signing with both hands, even though her arm is encased in plaster from shoulder to wrist, and her fingers are swollen to twice their normal size. I perch on the end of her bed.

"We'll be giving Brandy a break from chemo for a few weeks, Mom. But like I told you, we'll need to keep going for a good few months to make sure the cancer never comes back. Really exciting news, though. When the pathologist looked at where Brandy's cancer had been, he couldn't find a single cancer cell left alive."

Mom translates this latest news to Brandy. She turns her face towards me with a big grin.

By summer, I am making the trip to Columbus every few weeks, and Barbara sometimes stays at my apartment. We have found a psychologist couple, Joseph and Florence Zinker, at Cleveland's Gestalt Institute who specialize in couples work, including weekend workshops. It is my first experience of psychotherapy, and I warm to it quickly. I like the role-playing, Gestalt-style, and sharing our story with other couples. I am also thrilled I have been able to arrange with Ruth for Kate and George to come visit, and am busy exploring northern Ohio's attractions.

Three months into my new appointment, I accompany Sam to Chicago for a meeting of the Children's Cancer Study Group, one of two national organizations dedicated to treating children with cancer, constituted in 1967 by several university departments like our own. As we join the opening session, I am daunted by the sea of new faces. Sam introduces me to several men from West and East Coast institutions, whose names I promptly forget. I can identify the movers and shakers, though, and even follow how a national treatment protocol is put together. I sit in on a session of the leukemia committee, and see the results of the last ten years' research. I am astonished at how many patients have been enrolled, given the rarity of children's cancer compared to its adult counterpart.

Most therapies are designed as randomized clinical trials—something I've never seen constructed all the way from drawing board to clinical application. Promising new chemo drugs that have been already tested in a few larger centers are incorporated into these national trials. Newly diagnosed children are registered at a central statistical office, then randomly assigned to one or other treatment arm. Meaning that either they enter the standard treatment "arm," or they receive the new drug in addition to the standard, though neither family nor treating doctors know which arm the patient is on. The conduct of the trial is in the hands of the statisticians, to remove all possible bias from us physicians in judging if the new drug should be adopted permanently. Several statisticians are at this meeting, and they clearly play a critical part in ensuring a study's success.

On the final evening, a few of us gather to discuss creating a consortium of centers interested in stem cell transplants for children. There is only a handful of institutions represented, and no one seems eager to take the lead, though I get the strong sense Sam is pushing me. The two of us spend the trip back to Cleveland planning this new venture. Soon after our trip, I move into a bigger apartment in Cleveland Heights, with separate bedrooms for George and Kate, though they will only be staying a few weeks at a time. I am seeing Florence Zinker for personal counseling, and sobbing my way through each session. After putting me through psychological testing, she announces that I am clinically depressed—hardly earth-shattering news. She has me explore more non-work activities, so I acquire two cats, learn to cook healthier meals (never having cooked in my life), and start jogging with a colleague after work.

Ruth agrees to George and Kate coming for two weeks, so I quickly book my vacation. My conversations with them have been mostly brief answers to my queries about their day's activities, and their upcoming visit. But having them to myself is total joy. After some initial shyness, they are quickly competing for my attention, and telling me long tales of what they have been up to at home. We make many trips to an outdoor pool and to Cedar Point theme park, and stay up late for TV and countless food treats. When I finally get them into bed each night, I alternate which one to occupy for storytelling hour. After spending all my working days around ill children, having the exclusive company of my own two robustly healthy ones is a blessing beyond measure. As I put them on the plane home, I am choked with tears.

My patients mostly have cancers that I know all about from my work in London and Glasgow. But there are many black children with sickle cell disease, too, which I have never before encountered. They inherit two faulty genes that cause them to make the quite abnormal hemoglobin S. This creates sickle-shaped red cells during infections or just cold weather, so less oxygen can reach different body tissues and they often develop extreme pain resembling frostbite. Our only available treatments are opioid infusions, I.V. fluids, antibiotics, and blood transfusions which can shorten how long the current crisis lasts. I am on-call on my second New Year's Day in Cleveland when I meet Clayton—a fourteen-year-old who gets often readmitted. His pre-pubertal physique makes him look about ten, but there is no mistaking his teenage ways. He has an assortment of colorful T-shirts that hang to his knees, and an over-sized baseball cap permanently askew, with a shock of curly hair bunching out at the edges. A colorful tattoo covers one side of his neck, and another is tricked out on one arm.

When I approach his bed, he's pretty sleepy from his I.V. dilaudid. "Not too great a start to the new year, Clayton."

"Got that one right, doc. Sickle cell dizeeeze—curse of the Black Nation."

"You feeling any better? They told me they had trouble with your I.V. in the Emergency Room."

"Situation normal. My veins are shot from too many resident docs trying to stick 'em. I tell 'em which ones to go for, but they don't listen good. Figure they know better. Major pain."

"So how many times have you been in here?"

"Doc, I stopped counting way back. Closing in on a thousand, I guess. Belly and leg cramps mostly. Fevers, too. Or I can't catch my breath, 'cos of pneumonia. Sometimes they all come along at once. Crisis *doojoor*, you might say. Gets a lot worse now the weather's chillin'."

Sounds kind of proud of the whole thing—like he's out to beat all existing records.

"I guess you know a whole lot about it, then?"

"Yeah. They know me pretty well down in the E.R.—what to give me an' all. Sometimes they turn it around so I can go home, but mostly they stick me up here. Dilaudid two mills most times—mellows me out good. Can't take morphine, sets me to itching like red ants—and no way Benadryl cuts it. Been up in Intensive Care coupla times, too. My heart and lungs were fixing to give out."

"I don't think there's any danger of that this time, Clayton." But I am curious about just how many other drugs he is familiar with. "So what do they give you to go home on?"

"Oxy and Motrin mostly. Or Perc, maybe. Got in bad doodoo one time. Coupla new docs—they change 'em every year, you know that? So they hadn't checked my records, right? Figured I was a drug dealer, knowin' so much about things an' all. Saw my I.V. scars, so of course I had to be shootin' up." He smirks. "Guess the tats didn't help any. And Ma makin' sure I know *exactly* what's wrong with me, and *exactly* what they're supposed to do for it."

"I'll try to make sure that doesn't happen again, Clayton. They're making wristbands now—that could help. But your mom's right to make sure you know everything."

"I know it, doc. Thanks, okay?"

I continue on rounds, thinking of the life Clayton has been handed. He's in hospital more than he's home, let alone school, so he is getting himself some sort of education—but who needs life lessons like that? But I know he doesn't want my pity, any more than my cancer patients do. They are heroes all, and deserve to be recognized as such. I am humbled, and often uplifted, by having this chance to serve them. Being on-call is called being *on service* here—and what an apt description. Even when things get really hectic or aren't going well, being of service helps lift me out of my own black cloud state.

For the children with cancer the treatments are harsh, and their unwanted side effects many. But they are finite in length, and if we can ultimately cure them, after a few years they start living normal lives once more, with all its joys and challenges and accomplishments. It is quite different for Clayton. He isn't going to put his disease behind him before his dying day, which could come in his thirties or forties, or even earlier. Life expectancy for black men is significantly shorter than for whites, and sickle cell disease can take another huge chunk off. Does he ever reflect on this? Or does he just get on with living, hanging out with his buds, getting to school when he can, telling war stories about his latest hospital trip? Above all, he has a reputation for putting on a dauntless face and keeping his sense of humor intact, so he for sure doesn't need any gloomy docs around him.

I make my new year's resolution: I'll keep any downers of my own firmly under wraps, not let them interfere with bringing a positive spirit to work. Maybe it will lift a few others' spirits on a tough or gloomy day—the very least my patients deserve of me.

❧✿❧

Sam starts venting his feelings to me over department decisions being made behind closed doors. Even I am aware our chairman isn't winning any popularity contests, and several faculty members have left since I was hired. Then Sam announces out of the blue he wants a private chat with me. Am I going to get hauled over the coals for my poor teaching evaluations, or not yet garnering a nationally funded grant?

"So how are things, John?" he greets me. "It took you a while getting acclimated, but you're doing some great things. And how are things with you and Barbara?"

"Going great under the circumstances—living in different towns, I mean. Wish she could find permanent work here, but no luck so far."

I'm a bit taken back by the direction the conversation is headed, but his next words blow me away. "Well, I may have a solution. I've made a couple of trips to the University of Florida, and they want me to set up a brand new hem-onc program, hire faculty and shake things up down there. I want you to join me, set up a new transplant program. The department chair is all gung-ho. I even talked to him about Barbara—maybe creating a position for a departmental medical writer. Help faculty with grant writing, academic papers, that kind of thing. He's open to it, wants to meet you both. So what d'you think?"

I take a long moment to gather my thoughts. "Well, it sounds a very exciting offer. I'll need to talk to Barbara, of course, but I really appreciate your faith in me."

"Sure, take a few days, see what she says."

Too good to be true, not just his faith in me but having free rein setting up a stem cell unit. But Barbara has a secure job, and Florida isn't Ohio: just how much of a mid-westerner is she? But to my delight, she expresses huge excitement at exploring this new venture together.

Chapter 7: *GROUNDING*

The heat hits us as we step from the plane and make our way to the terminal. I am thrilled by my first glimpse of palm trees in the entranceway, set off by an array of tropical plants I can't put names to. Barbara is in high spirits, too, as we recapture our old joy and jokiness. We take a taxi to Mr. Wong's Chinese to meet Gerry Schiebler, the pediatric department's chair. There is an air of affability about the whole occasion as he introduces us to other faculty members. He seems more interested in getting up-to-date with Cleveland colleagues and exploring our family backgrounds than talking about our prospective jobs. He already has our C.V.'s, but makes no mention either of our credentials or his expectations. Lunch over, he drives us across University of Florida's expansive campus before touring us through Shands Hospital.

Our surroundings blur amidst countless lightning introductions. My afternoon passes in meetings with faculty, including Paulette Mehta, the only full-time pediatric hematologist, who is eager to have us join her. Barbara is whisked off by a realtor to look at houses that might appeal. Our appointments seem foregone, and the following weekend we celebrate my appointment as associate professor of pediatric hematology, oncology, and transplantation. Barbara is to become a full-time medical writer responsible for editing faculty and research fellows' papers and grant applications. I am already planning George and Kate's next trip, excited about exploring Disneyworld, Epcot, and the Florida beaches.

Back in Cleveland, I pack my worldly goods into my M.G.B., sell my few sticks of furniture, and bid goodbye to colleagues and friends. At my final visit to Florence, she repeats the psych tests and assures me I am in robust mental health. So much for culture shock! I secure my two cats in their carriers for my final trip to Columbus. Barbara, Julie and Amy have already loaded their car, and after coffee and mid-morning snacks we set out in convoy on the I-71 south across the Mason-Dixon line.

On my first ward round, I am welcomed by the residents with buttered scones and tea served in a china teapot. They clearly want me to feel at home, a far cry from the veiled hostility of their Cleveland counterparts. Sam and I meet our medical oncology colleagues, Roy and Jerry, to plan our new stem cell transplant unit. We decide to split the six beds between adult and child, expanding if we can keep a high occupancy. There are still few pediatric transplant units in the country, but Sam stresses what a source of revenue they can be. An average stay of six weeks readily racks up $100,000-plus, almost entirely covered by insurance or Medicaid. I find myself wondering if this should be our primary purpose, but keep the thought to myself. I am convinced from my Cleveland days that stem cell transplants are an exciting prospect for me, and for many future children under our care.

I set to work writing protocols for the hospital bioethics committee, working closely with Jerry, plus editorial input from Barbara, to hammer out criteria for transplanting patients with several hard-to-treat cancers. But if we thought we were ready to admit our first one, we hadn't reckoned with the committee's total ignorance of our therapies, and we find ourselves going line-by-line with them through each protocol. They are rightly concerned about the severe treatment toxicity—sometimes fatal—and the fact that we are charging patients for what some insurance companies claim are experimental therapies.

We finally get permission to go ahead, but an early patient brings the board's concerns right home. We had been treating three-year-old Kemal for advanced neuroblastoma, with painful deposits in his spine and pelvis and rosette-like clusters of cancer cells throughout his bone marrow. Two months of chemo puts Kemal into remission, but we know it is only a matter of time before the cancer shows up again. Our protocol calls for collecting large quantities of his marrow cells, now overtly free of neuroblastoma, for freezing in liquid nitrogen, as Roger had taught me in Cleveland. With Kemal fast asleep in the O.R., Sam and I set about collecting all the marrow we can from his hips. But when we estimate the number of healthy cells we have harvested, it barely exceeds the number we know we need to repopulate his blood.

And so it proves. We have to keep Kemal in isolation for almost six months as his blood counts inch towards safe levels. But his energy and appetite recover far faster, so our biggest problem is keeping him from breaking out of his cell. Mom spends day and night beside him, with brief respite when her husband or sister takes a shift. Kemal watches *The Muppet Movie* over and over, often into the early hours. By the time it's safe to discharge him, Mom estimates he has followed the antics of Kermit and Miss Piggy over five hundred times. In the alien world the little boy has been inhabiting, something about their lovable familiarity had become a source of comfort and reassurance.

Barbara and I move into a four-bedroom house in southwest Gainesville. Julie has turned eighteen and enrolls in the local community college, while fifteen-year-old Amy becomes a high school freshman. I love being around two healthy and lively teens after spending so much time with gravely ill ones. When George and Kate make their first Florida visit, our blended family relishes barbeques and frequent pool trips, along with Disneyworld and Epcot. But once I put them on a plane at Orlando airport, Barbara is unhappy with her job in the department and contemplating enrolling in the university's counseling education program. She starts drinking heavily at night, has trouble sleeping, and seems to falling into a permanent slump. She has yet to register with a doctor of her own, so I start prescribing Darvon for her insomnia and frequent migraines. From what I know of the drug, it is a benign pain-killer and sedative, and I have read no reports of its inclination towards dependency. I am filling prescriptions more often than is healthy, and Barbara has me call in refills at several different pharmacies, which should have tipped me off.

Amy takes a trip to visit her dad in Colorado over Christmas and decides to spend the year with him. Barbara and I start seeing another counselor, and for a time things go better. But after lengthy and difficult discussions towards the end of our first year in Gainesville, we decide on a trial separation. As I move my stuff into a rented house, I reflect on our three-year relationship. How I had fallen so heavily and deeply in love with her, precipitating my journey across the Atlantic, leaving behind not just Ruth but George and Kate. Only for Barbara and me to quickly run into trouble, first from my excessive dependence, then from preexisting problems of her own. Ruth still won't countenance the idea of divorce, which can't be helping things. Our counseling sessions end in squabbles or in Barbara shutting down, and now I am on my feet at work, and feeling better emotionally than I ever remember, my feelings for her are a mix of guilt and sadness. What started out so wonderfully has diminished barely to friendship.

Meanwhile, my work is proving all I had hoped. The stem cell unit has expanded to ten beds, and we are getting referrals from all over the Southeast. We have become a member of one of the two national consortiums of children's cancer centers, and at our second meeting I propose that we establish a transplant committee. Oncologists from eight other centers commit to joining, and I am asked to be chair. This will be a first: a national children's stem cell transplant consortium.

Gerry Schiebler lets me know I must sit the pediatric hematology-oncology boards, so I start to bone up on hematology, my longtime weakness. This leads to acquainting myself with the boys with hemophilia supervised by Paulette Mehta, and mostly treated by the residents in Emergency when they suffer a bleed into a joint. I realize I know little more about hemophilia than sketchy acquaintances back in Britain, going back to that house call on Mr. Deacon with Uncle Ken. If put to the test—which I certainly will be in the exam—I could say it's an inherited condition caused by a missing clotting factor—Factor VIII or IX—almost always affecting boys. But that is about the sum of my knowledge. I find out treatment hasn't changed much since the late 1950s, when donated and freshly frozen plasma started being infused to treat bleeding episodes, although it has mostly been replaced by a more concentrated factor VIII called cryoprecipitate. Early in Fall, 1981, Sam hands Paulette and me a copy of a newspaper report.

Rare Cancer Seen in 41 Homosexuals. Lawrence K. Altman, New York Times, July 3, 1981

Doctors in New York and California have diagnosed among homosexual men 41 cases of a rare and often rapidly fatal form of cancer. Eight of the victims died less than 24 months after the diagnosis was made. The cause of the outbreak is unknown, and there is as yet no evidence of contagion. But the doctors who have made the diagnoses, mostly in New York City and the San Francisco Bay area, are alerting other physicians who treat large numbers of homosexual men to the problem, in an effort to help identify more cases and to reduce the delay in offering chemotherapy treatment.'

None of the three of us realize it, but we are looking at the first description of A.I.D.S., manifesting as Kaposi's sarcoma.

"I don't know much about homosexuals in Florida," Sam comments, "but what I do know is a lot of these guys are regular blood donors at Pheresis

Centers, where they get paid—and we have one downtown. Bad news for our hemophiliacs, because the C.D.C. guys think this may be some weird infection from their plasma."

"So you mean all our hemophiliac boys run a risk every time we treat them?"

"Looks like it."

So it proves. I meet ten-year-old Gary in Paulette's clinic. He needs frequent cryo. infusions for swollen knees and ankles after trivial injuries. He had been admitted last week for bleeding starting under his tongue, which had become so hard to control it was obstructing his breathing. The idea of performing a tracheotomy to keep his airway open was too awful to contemplate, but was finally averted with continuous infusions around the clock for twenty-four hours. I introduce myself to Gary and his mom.

"I'm helping out Dr. Mehta today. I don't get to meet many guys like you, and I wanted to know more about how things are going. Did you get back to school yet, Gary?"

"No, I've been sick. Getting fevers and stuff."

"I'm really worried about him, doctor," his mother intervenes. "He didn't have a temperature when we checked into clinic, but it's up most evenings and all his muscles ache, and he can't keep anything down."

There isn't much to find on exam, but he certainly looks sick, and I suspect his liver is enlarged. I had just read about hepatitis C happening more often than expected in people needing frequent plasma infusions.

"Gary, I'm just going to chat to Dr. Mehta a minute. She knows you much better, so I want her to take a look at you too, okay?"

Mom looks relieved, and I don't blame her. Paulette has been looking after Gary since he was first diagnosed as an infant. I can almost hear her thinking, *What does this new guy know about anything?* She is not too wide of the mark.

"Mom, I think we should run a few tests," Paulette tells her after her own examination. "We've been seeing a few unusual infections in some of our boys. But it may be nothing to worry about at all."

A week later, Gary's results are back: his tests for hepatitis C are strongly positive. But before we can begin treatment, the little guy is overtaken by a far worse fate. He started having trouble breathing, which got worse fast. Despite being rushed to the I.C.U. to support his breathing, Gary succumbs to overwhelming pneumonia affecting both his lungs. The parents grant permission for autopsy, and the cause of his rapid demise is quickly identified: *pneumocystis* pneumonia, a fungal infection that especially affects people with weakened immunity.

"Some of those gay guys are getting the same thing," Sam says when we gather to talk about the situation.

"And I've just got a positive Hep C test back on another boy with severe hemophilia," Paulette adds. "It must be linked to the cryo infusions. I'm going to have our infectious disease docs screen all our boys to check their immune systems."

It turns out that many of them have dangerously low levels of T-lymphocytes (those derived from the thymus gland), putting them at risk for the same opportunistic infections affecting cancer patients with immunity weakened by chemo. It will be another two years before a virus is isolated in U.S. and French laboratories that is almost certainly the cause of what is widely called Acquired Immunodeficiency Syndrome.

We soon establish that H.I.V. is now affecting many hemophiliacs, including those at our clinic. We reserve cryo for particularly severe bleeds and only draw on Shands Hospital's pool of tried and tested donors. Then Paulette has more bad news.

"The Education Board is keeping two of our boys with Hep C out of school—just when they're gearing up for the new semester."

"But they're not a risk to other children, are they?"

"Absolutely not. And I don't think they'll make it to their teens, so why let them just wait for the other shoe to drop?"

"Well, I'm taking them to court," Sam announces, "get those boys back into school."

The case is heard at the local courts and the Education Board's case is upheld, the judge deciding there isn't enough evidence the children pose no risk to others. Sam persuades his lawyer to appeal, and the case is reheard in the state capital, Tallahassee. The appeals judge rules that the Education Board must let these boys back in school, "effective immediately." Also, any others with complications thought to arise from treatment must be allowed normal schooling, "if they are considered by their treating physicians to be healthy enough to benefit, without risk either to themselves or other children."

Sam celebrates by inviting us all to his house Friday night, where the wine and beer flow freely. But it's a hollow victory. In short order, several more boys succumb to severe infections, including three more pneumocystis pneumonias.

Ten centers are now entering patients onto our group transplant protocols, and I present our results and future plans to committees concerned with each individual cancer. But most of the over fifty centers have their own agendas, and are understandably reluctant to refer patients a long way from home for treatment both extremely aggressive and often unsuccessful in the long run. Childhood leukemia pioneer Don Pinkel from St. Jude's totally dismisses using stem cell transplants. "Exciting new agents are coming down the pike which we should all get behind. These transplanters are dead set on taking the heaviest of hammers to crack this nut . . . a practice whose time has gone!"

He carries a lot of weight, and St Jude's is not about to open its own unit. I get a similar reception from Ann Hayes, also at St. Jude's and chair of the neuroblastoma committee, when I present our results of autologous transplants for children with this disease. The statisticians back her up, dismissing our results as "merely anecdotal"—as though our brand new therapy counts for nothing. I hide my frustration while Sam, not given to such restraint, storms out of the meeting. A clear division has opened between our ten centers and those without stem cell units.

Back home, I start talking to some of our psychology faculty and get involved in studying knowledge and attitudes among peers of our cancer patients. I become a member of graduate student David Goodwin's Ph.D. committee exploring the quality of life of children with cancer, for which there is no good assessment scale. Since David's scale proves effective to assess both physical and emotional health in our patients, we bring it to the next gathering of our national consortium to try to get it adopted for widespread use.

Then another psychology colleague, Jim Rodrique, asks me about assessing anxiety in children coming into our transplant unit. "How well do you think their thoughts and feelings match those of their parents, John?" It takes my mind back to an eighteen-year-old Chinese boy, Joseph with thalassemia we had admitted to the unit. Could my psychology colleagues have got a good read on Joseph's mental state and that of his family?

Replacing the bone marrow cells of a person with thalassemia with those of a healthy donor can cure people of this ultimately fatal condition. In the

Northern Italian town of Pisaro over the past twenty years, many hundreds of children have been cured with stem cell transplants and are living the healthy lives of their friends and siblings. Joseph's family had immigrated to Miami from China's ancient capital, Xi'an, but Joseph had always been frail. A local hematologist diagnosed thalassemia and started monthly transfusions, then raised the possibility with his parents of stem cell transplantation. This becomes a certainty when blood tests on the family showed Joseph and six-year-old sister, Joy, share identical white cells—a one-in-four shot.

With their new-found knowledge—that this offered the only chance for Joseph to live a long life—the family traveled north to see me. One of our Taiwanese laboratory technicians acted as interpreter, because Dad spoke only rudimentary English and Mom apparently none. Unlike cancer patients, for whom the alternative is imminent death, Joseph could well live another ten years or more with transfusions alone, but he clearly understood this, while our interpreter seemed to think his parents understand all the dangers—that his life could be cut abruptly short from infection or other complications. It proved well nigh impossible to gauge their emotional state, because they remained deadpan throughout and asked almost no questions—quite unlike most of our parents. Joseph's father avoided my gaze as his small neat hand signed in triplicate on the bottom line of each of the consent forms I handed him.

Clearly communication during the arduous time ahead for Joseph would be a big challenge. But the die was cast. A week later, we filled Joseph's body with the super-high chemo doses needed to prepare the ground to establish Joy's healthy cells inside his now empty marrow spaces. While sister Joy dreamt the morning away, we drew off large quantities of marrow cells from her hip bones with our giant 50-cc syringes, and infused them through the catheter inserted into Joseph's heart. No one knows exactly how these donated cells know to "home" on their newly-adopted marrow cavity. But take a small sample from a patient three weeks later, and like as not you will see these immigrant cells starting to fill up the spots so recently emptied out by our chemo. One of life's lovely mysteries: every cell knows its place. The two children accepted the whole thing as an adventure, but their parents had entered almost blindly into this strange world of high-tech medicine. How much did they really grasp of what their son was facing? Impossible to know.

The transplant behind us, the intensive nursing began to pilot Joseph through the perilous waters before Joy's cells started multiplying within him.

Until these seedlings began to put forth their shoots into his bloodstream, Joseph would need a constant supply of antibiotics, red cells, and platelets. With no platelets to block the holes, he could bleed freely inside and out. Our blood bank had a well-oiled machine for platelet donation and a flock of willing donors; many of our unit's staff and our university's fifty-thousand students are regulars. Even so, give enough platelet transfusions, and like as not you run up against the body's resistance—a situation when only those most closely matched with the recipient will produce a brief blip in the platelet count.

Race compounds this. Finding matches for ethnic minorities is much tougher, because white cell and platelet types differ with race. So it proved with Joseph. Two weeks out, his body was devouring platelets faster than we could pour them in—and we had run out of donors. The only one who could stem the tide was off-limits: six-year-old Joy's tiny veins could never handle our fat fourteen-gauge needles.

I got the call at five o'clock one early-July morning. Joseph's platelet count had hit an all-time low, despite our scouring the nation for compatible donors. Joseph's nurse, Bonnie, had picked up daunting signs: a slow but steady rise in blood pressure and accompanying fall in pulse rate. One cause for these changes is rising pressure inside the brain. Could Joseph be having an insidious cerebral hemorrhage? Though he'd had no major bleeding episode, there had been telltale signs for the past few days: a blossoming of bruises over pressure areas when lying too long in one position, a scattering of blood blisters in his mouth, bursts of nose bleeds controllable only with wads of gauze. I scurried to my car under one of Florida's midsummer cloudbursts, willing myself not to speed on the wet streets. By the time I got there, things had deteriorated. When Bonnie had tried rousing Joseph, he had complained of pressure in his head, then started to ramble and slur his speech. His pulse rate was fifty and falling, blood pressure 150 over 100, and his body was a mass of bruises, most of them fresh.

Things moved fast. We rushed him out of the unit into the elevator and down to X-ray, where the on-call technician whisked him under the C.A.T. scanner. Watching the screen, we could see blood trickling into his lateral ventricles. By the time he was back upstairs and someone had got his parents to the scene, Joseph was slipping into coma. His last words on earth were a little song, as though offering solace to his family, to us, to himself.

Dad eyed the whole scene stony-faced, while Mom stifled her sobs. I struggled to clarify what had transpired, but no interpreter had been located, and Joseph could no longer explain. They struggled to hide any exhibition of public sorrow, but Joy, unschooled in Eastern culture, had no such inhibitions. Grasping what was happening, she pushed herself into her brother's isolation room, crying freely: "Why must my brother die?" Her high sing-song voice quavered like a hermit thrush. Then, "Is he an angel yet?"

Bonnie, standing beside her, stretched out her arms: "Do you want to say goodbye to him?"

"Can I listen to him with the steth-o-scope?" Pronouncing the word with precise articulation, syllable by syllable. But her father grabbed her and drew her back. Our Taiwanese lab technician told me later the parents probably held deep cultural beliefs that direct physical contact with their dying boy risked holding his soul forever in this world. They sat mute and apart, several feet from his bed. I could do no more for Joseph, and his parents were utterly remote from more explanation or solace. So Joy let me lead her by the hand down the passageway to our art room. Settled at the table, she started to paint, first my portrait, then her brother's, crying every few minutes, then dipping her brush into the poster paint to splash more colorful daubs, before pausing to weep some more. At seven o'clock, as the sunlight peeked through the high window, it came to Joy how hungry she was, so we rode the elevator to the hospital cafeteria for an early breakfast. She munched her way through a brimming bowl of Fruit Loops, then scrambled eggs on toast, washed down with a carton of Choco-milk. From time to time, she paused to shed more tears, which did nothing to mar her appetite.

Joseph died while she was putting the finishing touches to her portraits. Her parents hadn't let her say farewell to him, so as the family took its leave, clutching three paper bags holding Joseph's earthly possessions, Joy made a formal ritual of saying, in her thrush's voice, goodbye to me instead. It was three hours since I had got the first alarm call. Paint was still sticky on each of her finger pulps.

We never heard from the family again, and my attempts to reach them by phone went unanswered. I wrestled with whether we were right to go ahead with the transplant, when we had so little handle on the parents' level of understanding or true feelings about exposing their son to what proved such a rapidly fatal attempt at treatment. I talked to my psychologist friend, Jim Rodrigue, about whether he thought a family's level of understanding and emotional state should ever influence our decision whether or not to use such a perilous form of treatment. His answer was appropriately judicious.

"John, it will always be a matter of weighing the very real risks against the possible benefits. It's a whole lot easier when a patient has a cancer that is almost certainly going to kill him or her quickly without the transplant. But when it comes to Joseph, who you say might have lived another ten or more years? Well, I'm just glad I wasn't the one who had to make that decision."

Then I meet Ed—or rather make his reacquaintance. At eighteen, he had been one of the most compliant adolescents I've cared for in twenty years. His cancer—non-Hodgkin lymphoma —had started in his pelvis, pressing on his left kidney and transverse colon, and clumps of malignant cells were strewn throughout his bone marrow. He had sailed through six hefty rounds of chemo and looked on the road to cure, making the dean's list in our pre-med program, then switching to clinical psychology for his Ph.D. Then five years on, almost to the day, his cancer recurs. At twenty-three, Ed is his own man, and decides it's time for the medical oncologists to take over from us peds guys. He makes it through four more rounds of chemo, plus a couple of thousand rads of irradiation to his belly. Hardly plain sailing this time, but he emerges in total remission once more. All of us agree, Ed is heading for a stem cell transplant.

At our weekly meeting, Hal, the oncologist on duty this month, announces his plans. "Allogeneic transplant's not an option—no matched donor. But we checked Ed's marrow yesterday—not a cancer cell in sight. I'm thinking to freeze his stem cells next week, then bring him straight into the unit. Strike while the iron is hot."

But Ed has been keeping in touch with me—and sharing a very different scenario.

"There's a wrinkle," I tell Hal. "He maybe didn't mention it, but he's planning on getting married. This coming weekend."

"Hell, he kept that close to his chest." Hal looks disconcerted for ten seconds. "So can't he rearrange his schedule?"

"No, Hal. He's been figuring out the odds against coming out of our unit alive. With his immunity shot to hell after ten rounds of hefty chemo plus that abdominal R.T. under his belt already, then wiping everything out before the transplant. . . . Well, that's the very reason they've moved up their wedding date."

I let this sink in. We've all had our private conversations. Knowing what we know, would we put ourselves through it? Our partners? Our children? Six weeks-plus of miserable toxicity, twelve months or more to recover to full functioning. In Ed's case, given all the therapy he has already come through, there is a real likelihood of permanent damage to his liver, lungs, kidneys, psyche—you name it.

Hal's pause lasts a little longer. I don't say it out loud, but he had better be ready for a tough "informed consent" session. For Ed taking charge. We sometimes pay lip service to that word—autonomy. To Ed, though, it really does mean, "*You* don't decide, *I* do. No imposing your own opinions about what's best for me." He's not just smart, he's feisty. He'll want chapter and verse on what he is in for—complete with every stat Hal can come up with. Ed knows his Nuremberg Code—and all those bioethical issues our review board presses on us with every protocol we submit.

"Well, we sure can't afford to wait too long," Hal says finally. "Surely he'll see that. How long a honeymoon are they planning?"

"You'd have to ask him. Why don't you just plan to hold off a couple of weeks?"

So a month later, Hal sits down to consent Ed in our social worker, Penny's, office. Later, Penny gives me the scoop. How Ed and his brand new bride, Alice, had listened intently while Hal had run through the five-page consent form and finished his spiel. Then Ed had pressed his oncologist on the exact risks of not emerging alive. How big was the danger of fatal infection? How about long term damage? What about fathering children with Alice? He had finished by requesting copies of every research study Hal had to back up his recommendations. Hal had hurriedly set up a second meeting, this time armed with even more research articles and citations on stem cell transplant for relapsed and heavily pre-treated non-Hodgkin's lymphoma.

Penny must have been taking notes of her own—she has this second session down pretty much verbatim. Once again, Ed had listened carefully, then plunged Hal into uncharted waters.

"What exactly is your nursing coverage at night?"

"Well, I'd need to check on that."

"Do any of you transplant docs sleep in the unit?"

"Er, no. But the on-call attending is always a phone call away. Twenty-four-seven."

"You've got dedicated resident coverage at night?"

"Pretty close. There's a senior resident covering the oncology floor, with ready access to the unit. And the I.C.U. guys are just three floors above."

"Tell me how folks deal with living twenty-four hours day-in, day-out under your laminar air flow set-up? For six weeks, maybe longer?"

"Yeah, it's tough." Hal doesn't come up with anything more on that one.

"How about privacy? How much can Alice and I expect? We wouldn't be crazy about docs and nurses wandering in and out at all hours without a by-your-leave."

This is way outside Hal's purview—and he isn't about to quiz Ed about exactly what conjugal rights he plans to exercise during his prolonged spell of close to zero white cells and platelets.

"Er, I'd have to talk to our nurse manager about that."

Penny pauses to grin wryly. "It was getting pretty tense in there, John. Ed had all these questions down pat. But I sensed the fear right close under the surface that he was trying to keep from Alice. With her set to burst into tears at any moment. Meanwhile, Hal was getting more and more frustrated, and beginning to show it. He's just not used to this kind of interrogation, and I don't think he was getting it that this wasn't just Ed wanting every last clinical fact. A lot of it was simply cover-up for the emotional turmoil he was in."

Ed had wrapped up the session by shaking Hal's hand and thanking him for all the trouble he'd gone to, then announced that he was going to interview us peds guys, too.

"It's not that I don't have every faith in your team. It's just I've known those docs a whole lot longer. And I want to be sure you're all on the same page."

He interviews Sam first, then gets around to me, with Alice again sitting beside him on the couch in Penny's office. We chitchat about the wedding, and their honeymoon plans once everything is behind them. I feel the atmosphere ease as Ed and Alice let themselves glimpse beyond the ordeal ahead, contemplate their future together. I finally cut to the chase.

"Ed, Alice, I don't think you want me to snow you with any more facts and figures. You've had a fistful already. But maybe just a bit more about what to expect if you do decide to go ahead. There'll be some real rough patches, for sure. It's something I wouldn't want my own family to have to go through. But I know you, Ed—and I know you can do this. Of course there are options—you don't have to put yourself and Alice through it. Maybe you want to talk some more about those options?"

"We understand all that, doc. Essentially, we could buy some time with lighter therapy. But we know full well how that would end up in the end."

We chat back and forth for another thirty minutes, Penny adding her own comments about how others get through it, some things she knows can help. I do a lot more listening than talking. Then Ed sits back, his arm around Alice, and looks full on at me.

"Thanks. You didn't pull punches but you sound pretty hopeful. Gives me the confidence I've been needing. I'm ready to sign."

The day he enters the unit, Ed gives our head nurse copies of his own documents. His power of attorney and personal directive, both naming Alice, and their typed-up personal privacy requests.

"Look, I know your nurses have to check on me at least once a shift. Absolutely fine. And if any staff decide there's a problem, then I'm cool with whatever they need to do. But Alice will be there with me twenty-four-seven—and she's seen me through plenty already. I think she is going to know right off if I'm in any kind of trouble."

I check in with them before I head out, trying to picture for myself what it has to be like, this time-bomb of an illness. It could have so easily carried him off already, and now here they are, putting themselves in the hands of nursing team number three. Ed had got to know all our peds unit nurses and treated them as buddies. Then he'd come to trust the oncology nurses while he was going through his last tough set of treatments. But the transplant unit is a whole different ballpark. It rates its intensive care designation for good reason, and Ed will have to take on faith this new staff's competence or otherwise in his life-or-death ordeal. No wonder he wants control over *something*. Would I ever have got this far?

In the end, he comes through with flying colors, almost breezing through his post-transplant recovery phase. Though the usual six weeks had stretched out to eight, and "breeze" hardly captures life in that goldfish bowl: the inevitable plague of excruciating mucositis, skin peeling off in raw patches, long days of nausea, diarrhea, and fever. The near-solitary confinement, days stretching into weeks. Ed's and Alice's emotions seesawing between boredom and nameless dread. But six months later, he shows up in my office looking the very picture of health: back to his fighting weight, cheeks aglow, scalp a mass of fine dark curls.

"You look fantastic, Ed. Married life sure suits you!"

"Two hundred and fifty days today. But don't let my looks fool you. I thought once I got out of the unit I'd get my life straight back into the fast lane. Wrong! Hardly a day I don't wake from some bad dream, scared like a baby the cancer is back. Take three-hour naps after lunch. Barely enough energy for classes, let alone my Master's thesis. Anyway, that's what I want to talk to you about. Alice thinks getting my teeth into it would be good therapy—a whole sight better than watching T.V. movie reruns. So I'm gearing up to put my proposal together. I want to look at what I've learned from all I've been through. I think I've got some stuff to say that others could benefit from."

"That's for sure. So—what have you got in mind?"

"Well, maybe it's good this whole experience is fresh in my mind. In my psyche, really. I want to hone in on those informed consent sessions." He grins. "I know I was a bit of an outlier, interviewing each one of you guys, pitching a zillion curved balls before I'd sign the go-ahead. Most patients don't push it the way I did, right?"

"Right—most are too scared. Find it easier to put it back on us docs, trust us we're doing the right thing for them."

"And maybe we don't want to risk making you mad, so you won't give us all your care and attention. But you know, I used to sit there in front of you guys with my long list of questions, and pretty soon it got harder and harder to hold onto the answers. Let alone take anything useful away from them."

"Well, the bioethics board certainly insists we hit you with every possible side effect."

"That's just it. What research I *have* uncovered suggests you docs have little idea how much your patients *can* take in. Before we shut down and stop listening, I mean."

"I wonder about it every time I sit down with my consent forms. How much does this person really need to know? And how much do they want to? So you have something in mind?"

"Yes. I want to look at our whole decision-making when we do get sick. And especially how our emotions affect it. I talked to some of the Psych faculty, they think it has great research potential. And I'm clearly the right one to do it. I've thought a lot about those consent sessions. Why couldn't I say 'enough already, just get on with it?' About drove Hal crazy. And I'm positive my comfort level affected how much I could take in of what I was hearing.

"You docs are so different in how you relate to your patients. Some relaxed and comfortable, like you have all the time in the world, always good eye contact, listening as much as talking. Really responding to the questions you're posed, rather than spouting from some prepared script. But others can hardly bring themselves to sit down, then they fill the air with technical stuff. Giving off all these non-verbal cues when they're getting antsy, or impatient. Folding their arms across their chest, avoiding my eye, shuffling papers around—just wanting to get done with the whole thing. Enough to trigger anyone's anxiety. My theory is anxious people quickly stop taking anything in, but this just hasn't been tested empirically."

He cuts to the chase. "Okay. So I want to look at how these physician cues influence patient decision-making. Not just how Jo or Joanna patient *feels* afterwards, but how much they take in and *understand*. I want to set up mock patient-doctor interviews, and study how varying the way the doc acts affects the patient's response. See if my theory bears out in a valid research setting." He stops and beams at me. "You've done quite a bit of acting, haven't you?"

"Now, how d'you come to know that?"

"Oh, you mentioned it one time. Told me how sitting and talking with patients is like role-playing. And you had to learn to play that part well, just as an actor on stage has to. That this doesn't get the attention it deserves—how non-verbal cues can affect doctor-patient rapport. So supposing I created a situation where you had to report to patients some ambiguous and scary X-ray findings. You'd have to do this with two groups, but vary your *affect*—your demeanor—in how you behaved in their presence, and in the way you reported these X-rays. Okay?"

"But surely there'd be a huge ethical problem, Ed. From what I'm hearing, you're going to have me tell real live patients the same information, but change the way I do it each time?"

"No, no, nothing like that. You know what an analog study is?"

"Try me."

"It's when you replicate a real-life situation under artificially controlled conditions. It gets us psych folks around a bunch of problems the bioethics board would shoot us down for. I plan to recruit as many women as I can with higher than normal risks of breast cancer. A family history, or early menarche; a history of benign breast lumps; or being on menopausal estrogen. Then I'd film two separate videos of you presenting the results of a recent mammogram report that is purportedly their own. Our consent form would explain they were taking part in a completely simulated research study—I don't think too many women would balk at that.

"The important thing is, the mammogram report would show *ambiguous* results. And it would include the same information each time, with a clear recommendation for further testing. Then I'd randomly assign the women to two groups. The first would watch a video of you appearing tense and anxious as you read and interpret the results. With the second, you'd do the same thing but seem relaxed and confident. The single difference in the script would be that you'd say "I'm worried" several times in the first tape, and "I'm not worried" several times in the second. In addition, you'd introduce lots of non-verbal "worried" and "not worried" cues to match your words. What d'you think?"

"Sounds like fun. What are you planning to measure?"

"Several things. We'd use established tests to get an immediate record of how anxious the women were after watching the tape. Then we'd assess how medically serious the subjects viewed their situation, using a nine-point scale. Lastly, we'd measure how much factual information the two groups had *understood* of everything you'd presented, using a seven-point questionnaire of their recall and understanding."

"So if you find differences, it would have implications for training us docs, right? About the importance of how we deliver ambiguous information to our patients. And I don't have to tell you, medicine's chock full of ambiguities."

"So you're up for it?"

"You bet. Thanks for asking me."

Making the two films proves easy, and Ed recruits forty suitably at-risk subjects through ads posted around the health center and the city. Another six months, and I'm sitting in on one of the psychology department's research seminars where Ed is presenting his results for the first time. He's in his Sunday best—I've never seen him so dressed up. He sets the scene, then gets to the meat of his findings.

"You'll see there's a striking difference between the two groups of women in their anxiety measures. Those watching the 'worried' videotape had significantly faster heart rates both during and right afterwards. And they also scored significantly higher on the state-anxiety scale than the 'non-worried' group. The 'worried' watchers also saw the situation as significantly more serious than the 'non-worried' watchers. Last—and perhaps the key difference. The group of women watching the 'non-worried' physician got significantly more answers correct on our questionnaire testing their understanding than those watching the 'worried' tape."

No one is left in any doubt. It goes without saying that accurate information is vital for patients to make their best decisions. But *how* the doctor presents that information seems to matter even more. One of the senior faculty pipes up.

"Jaw-dropping stuff, Ed. And this isn't even real life, far from it. You've got a doctor on a videotape simulating the whole thing, with twenty women watching simultaneously. But by the end of it, the 'worried' watchers aren't fit to decide on Corn Flakes or Wheaties for breakfast! Beautiful work."

A year later, Ed presents me with a copy of an article he has just published in a prestigious psychology journal, under a suitably scholarly title twenty-one words long. "Analogue," "Physician affect," and "Subject recall" all feature prominently.

I get an invitation to join our hospital bioethics board, and at my first meeting the chairman takes me aside over coffee before bringing the meeting to order.

"I'm really glad you've joined us, John. These protocols you're sending are proving tough to get consensus on. Some seem to think you guys have even forgotten the Nuremberg Code. And these kids, especially the youngest ones, don't have any say in what you do to them. None of that vital autonomy granted to adults. I tell you, pediatric ethical issues are the worst."

I have a flashback to my *ad hoc* bioethics committee last week in our ward conference room to decide on ten-year-old Kyle's fate. Kyle had developed his cancer a year before. A sarcoma arising deep in his belly, it had responded minimally to different chemo regimens, and our best next step wasn't clear even after considerable discussion. Should we try increasingly experimental therapies, hoping for a breakthrough, or just let nature take its course? Sensing strong differences of opinion between my colleagues and perhaps between staff and family, I had gathered a small group to seek consensus, including Kyle's parents. An unconventional step, but parents have every right to be in on any debate when there are no black-and-white answers.

As we settle around the table, one of our research fellows, who has taken on Kyle's case as a personal mission, presents chapter and verse of a chemo regimen that is a new departure. She quotes from the most recent journal report: "reportedly shows promise in similar cases, albeit the follow-up on the patients averages only three months." Early days, indeed, to make any strong claims, and she acknowledges that the patients had spent long spells in hospital recovering from side effects, but as I look around the room, I sense consensus between us and Kyle's parents. Even though Kyle's outlook is bleak, this new experimental treatment is worth a try. Surely better than watching him die without all of us fighting for his life. In the end, though, ten-year-old Kyle makes his own decision. When I sit down with him and his parents an hour later, he starts quizzing me.

"Will it make me better?"

"Well, I can't promise that, Kyle. But I think there's a chance. A good one."

"Will I have to stay in the hospital?"

"Yes, buddy. For a few days, maybe a bit more." I'm hedging, not holding his direct look. That look that tells me he thinks I'm full of shit. I have no idea how long he will be hospitalized each time, because we have no experience with this new drug combination, and no way to know how he will respond in his already weakened state, given his cancer had almost laughed off our front-line therapy. I have also, conveniently, not let him know we are planning six consecutive drug courses if his cancer does respond.

Kyle looks at his mother, then back at me. "What you did before, that didn't work, did it? None of it. You told me."

He's got me. All of us. Kyle breaks the silence.

"Anyway, I want to go home. I'm not staying in this hospital anymore."

Something tells me he's not ready for further argument or attempts at persuasion. So has he reached the age of consent? Far from it. But the whole concept of legal age of consent for minors has gone straight out the window. I am face-to-face with a young man who has aged ten more years over the past four months of futile treatment that has done little except cause horrendous side effects. Doped up with drugs for pain and nausea caused in equal part by the cancer and the chemo, he's lost twenty pounds, and hardly been home, let alone to school or to hang out with his buddies. His dad speaks up.

"Fair enough, pal, you've given it your best shot. Maybe it's time you had a spell at home, so you can do stuff you've been missing out on." He directs his son's same direct gaze at me. "Right, doc?"

I reach my decision. "Yes, I think you're right. I can give you a good supply of medicines so Kyle doesn't hurt too much. Give him a bit of an appetite, help him sleep, too. We can arrange for some home nursing visits—we can talk about all that."

As I'm saying this, I'm aware my medical colleagues might take issue with this whole decision-making process. Do Kyle's parents, does Kyle himself, have the right to decide his fate like this? To "give up" on fighting for the life of this child, this minor? What if the lawyers want to step in, insist that letting a ten-year-old refuse possibly life-saving treatment is indefensible? Well, there *are* no lawyers present, and I'm not about to summon one.

Kyle lives on for another three weeks at home. The parents welcome the visits of our local hospice team, and they are with him the night he falls asleep for the last time. I make one home visit—to their small town 60 miles south of Gainesville—and keep in touch by phone. It takes me back thirty years to nocturnal vigils with Uncle Ken to the bedsides of miners, sitting beside teenage sons and daughters. Kyle's death seems at least peaceful and pain-free. His family accepts all that happened over the past months, and in time my colleagues seem to as well. Ten-year-olds can sometimes defy the statutes of the law and make their own life-and-death decisions.

This is the last stanza of "Consensus and Consent," a requiem I wrote for Kyle.

. . . Kyle, consulted about testing such terra incognita, and infirma,
says: No, I want to stay home. *So be it. He has, we all concede,*
reached the age of consent, whenever that may be.

The American Association of Pediatric first published its policy on the legal concept of informed consent in 1976. Then, in 1984, the association's committee on bioethics fully recognized that minors, "especially those aged 14 or older may have as well-developed decisional skills as adults," and we should always seek to include them in our decision-making. But I am unaware of guidelines about how these complexities should be presented to the young ones themselves. But their refusal or consent may well be not only ethically but legally binding. So once all the facts are clear to everyone, ethics—in medicine as in life—comes down to acting on your best judgment and conscience.

But what about couples who are by the letter of the law children themselves—under eighteen—when they have their own child? Brendan and Malila were aged sixteen when son Hughie was born. When he was four months old, Brendan felt a lump in Hughie's buttock while soaking him in the tub. Their doctor referred him to our pediatric surgeons, who biopsied it next morning. I learned the same day that it was cancerous—a sarcoma, like Kyle's—and went to visit the family. Malila was tucked up in a bed next to the crib where Hughie lay sleeping peacefully. It turned out she'd had stomach cramps and been throwing up, so she was now a patient herself on our pediatric ward.

"Brendan, Malila, I'm a specialist who looks after children like yours. And I'm sorry to say I've got some bad news about your little one. There is no easy way to tell you this, but Hughie has a kind of cancer."

Silence, a few eternities long. Then Malila starts screaming, while Brendan stares stupefied at his sneakers. As the cries subside to whimpers, I judge it time to press on.

"We don't know why this happened, but we do know it's nothing you did, or didn't do. That's for darn sure. And we have these special drugs we can give Hughie to shrink it right down. Chemotherapy, we call it—chemo, for short."

I go on talking, but Brendan has switched off and is busying himself with the vomit bowl as Malila starts throwing up again. I'm back early next day with my stack of papers to explain our treatment plan and get their consent. But I have grave misgivings about how well these two are going to grasp the intricacies of large-scale national drugs trials.

"Brendan, Malila, I've got to tell you everything about this treatment, so you both understand and agree to it. You see, it's urgent to get started, but the drugs can do a lot of bad things, as well as good." I shuffle my papers. "We call this document here a consent form. We can't start anything till you sign it, showing you agree with everything I've told you. People under eighteen can't usually sign, but we make exceptions when you're the parents. You're what the lawyers call emancipated minors."

Brendan looks like he's trying to grab at my words, but I suspect they're sailing past him, gone somewhere where he can't hold onto them.

"Hughie's cancer is very rare, and I'm sorry to tell you, not everyone makes it even with our best medicines. So we're always finding new ones, trying to make things better. We have this system for testing each new drug by adding it to our usual ones. It's kind of an experiment, okay?"

Brendan suddenly realizes I've stopped talking and am waiting on his answer.

"Guess so."

"So you see, Hughie might get just the usual drugs, or he might get a brand new one in addition. A computer decides it—sort of like tossing a coin."

I hand a wad of papers to Brendan, hesitate before offering Malila a second wad. She's squirming and dry-heaving into the bowl clutched between her knees.

"That's cool, I'll go over it with her later."

Brendan doesn't add that reading isn't Malila's strongest suit—I only discover this later. I start going page-by-page, word-by-word, over each section, spelling out the drug names, along with all the scary stuff they could possibly do to Hughie. Brendan hangs in for most of one sheet before looking like his brain has turned upside down. I flip over several pages to a chart laying out the whole treatment plan in the form of arrows, bold capital letters, and stick figures.

"I think this will help. Each letter stands for a drug in our treatment plan."

Brendan eyeballs the chart. "So—these M.'s and C.'s, and more M.'s, that's what Hughie's going to get, right?"

"That's it."

"Then these two—V. and D.—after that?"

"Right again!"

"And maybe he'll get this one too. This T. here. Or maybe not. That's where the coin tossing comes in."

"You're catching on, Brendan!"

"So when do we get to take him home?"

"Ah, not for a good few weeks. You heard me tell you about all those things that can happen to him?"

"He'll lose his hair, right?"

We both glance at Hughie's beautiful coal-black curls.

"Well, not right off. But it's these other things . . ."

"Yeah, yeah. We gotta watch him for fevers. Sore butt. Nosebleeds. All that stuff."

"You're doing great. Seems like you know something about all this."

"Seen it on T.V., about this woman. These drugs, they work?"

"Oh yeah, they work."

I notice Malila is snoring quietly, left thumb wedged between her lips. Hughie is blissed out in la-la land, face pressed against the crib bars, as Brendan signs the triplicate copies of the consent form. How much Dad really understands about randomized clinical trials I'll never know. We get the chemo up and running early that afternoon, and I check back in with the family before I leave. I pause at the door of the room as I take in the sounds of altercation. A woman perhaps in her forties, presumably a grandma, is clutching what looks like the signed consent form in her fist and waving it at Brendan.

"What's all this shit they're doing to him, Bren? You understand what's going on? Well, I understand full well. They're *experimenting* on him."

"Wait, Mom . . ."

"Look here. Look, where it says these drugs can give him seizures. And heart troubles. You don't get over heart troubles. You understand that, boy?"

Brendan is slowly unwrapping himself from where he'd been spooned against Malila's back. He props himself up on the side of the bed to meet his mom's glare.

"And what's this about tossing a coin? This part about a computer deciding things? They're not tossing no coin over my grandson." She shakes the plastic bottle hanging above Hughie's crib like she's all set to rip it free of the tube vanishing beneath the big bandage around his leg. "So what's in here? Poisons, right? You understand all this stuff, do you, Brendan?"

"Sure I do, Mom."

"Okay, *Doctor* Marshall, so you tell me what's in this bottle?" She spits out the words, and Brendan has a hard time cutting her off before she winds herself up again.

"Now just cool it, Mom, okay? And don't mess with that. They got the drugs in there to kill his cancer. I signed him up for it."

"You can't do that, boy! You're under age. Only grown-ups can sign for that stuff."

The triumph in her voice is all too evident. But now Brendan faces her full on.

"Yeah, I can. Doc said so. We're his mom and dad, so they make exceptions."

With that, he starts right into his litany, snapping it out super-fast as though worried he'll forget something vital.

"He's getting M, then C, then three more M's. Then he'll get V and D. That's the drugs—there's a picture in there shows you. And his hair will fall out but not yet awhile, and he'll likely get fevers and we'll have to get his blood checked a bunch, and they'll test his heart and kidneys—and he's not going to get no seizures, they just have to put that in."

He stops to take a long breath. Grandma is clearly silenced by her son's speech. She blinks, half-turns, and spots me.

"This is the doc that talked to us, Mom."

Brendan looks relieved that support has arrived.

"You read all that stuff, son?"

"Doc did. I just followed along."

"So what about her?" glancing at Malila. "She read it?"

"She was asleep. He only needed one of us to sign."

Grandma drops into the space on the bed that Brendan has just vacated. She looks at her son a long frowning moment. Then the frown transforms to joy.

"I'm proud of you, Bren. You catch on real fast when you've a mind. And Hughie, he's blessed to have you for his dad."

The computer assigned Hughie to the standard treatment arm, and he sailed through his whole protocol with no major setbacks. When our surgeon came to operate to remove any residual tumor, there was none to be found. But the whole thing left me wondering about informed consents, and how meaningful they could possibly have been to Bren and Malila.

≽❀≼

I make a trip back to England for an oncology conference, and spend several days with now ten-year-old George and almost eight-year-old Kate. On Sunday at London Zoo we survey the giraffes, penguins, and all species in between before feasting on the Victoria Station Hotel carvery. All three of us tuck into mounds of roast lamb, beef and turkey, plus all the trimmings, followed—in George's case—by apple pie topped with two scoops of ice cream. I feel proud to be maintaining this close relationship with my children at such distance. Between my visits to Britain and theirs to me, we've been getting together several times a year, although after almost seven years of separation, Ruth still dismisses any discussion of divorce. Back in Gainesville, I experience an unfamiliar feeling of homecoming, realize I'm becoming more and more comfortable in my ex-pat persona.

My adult oncology colleagues get interested in developing protocols based on the ones we're using for transplanting children with forms of acute leukemia and lymphoma they see less often. Neuroblastoma is almost unheard of in grown-ups, so our promising results in this hitherto incurable disease catch their attention. Much of our success with children seems to come from how an eight-year-old can tolerate the massive chemo doses far better than a fifty-eight-year-old. Their greater responsiveness and resilience lets us pediatricians lay claim to some leadership, at least for cancers common to all ages. I get invited to join a multicenter consortium of transplant oncologists where I will be the sole voice speaking for pediatricians. We've been using stem cell transplants in children with advanced neuroblastoma for four years at seven centers, and have a hundred-plus cases to report on. Close to half those transplanted after initial chemo are still in remission—far better than any non-transplant regimen has ever achieved. But given the entrenched attitude of many pediatric cancer centers—either adamantly opposed, or else convinced transplant is the only way forward—the notion of a randomized trial, the gold standard for newly tested treatments, is a non-starter.

My growing interest in child psychology takes an unexpected turn. On New Years Eve, 1984, I'm at a party on a farm south of Gainesville, and shortly before midnight catch sight of a blond woman drinking punch at a trestle table under the stars. I quickly discover Sheila is another pediatric psychologist, or—as she quickly corrects me—a child psychologist, a professor on sabbatical from Oregon Health Sciences University.

"*Child* psychologists work entirely with physically healthy children with emotional ('acting out' or 'acting in') problems," she adds. "*Pediatric* psychologists spend their time wrestling with psychological issues arising in children with physical illness. I steer well clear of all those sick kids on the inpatient wards."

Within a few minutes we realize everyone is gathered around the two of us. As voices rise to greet the New Year with "Auld Lang Zyne," our host announces it is also my new friend's fortieth birthday. The following week, I find out exactly why Sheila makes a point of avoiding the wards when I invite her to make rounds with me. We are joined by our fellows, residents, and social worker, Anne, and I'm emerging from my first patient's room to find Sheila has disappeared. Anne draws me aside.

"I think the atmosphere was a bit overwhelming for Dr. Eyberg, John. Can you break away a minute?"

I follow Anne back down the passage. Sheila is stretched out on the floor outside the ward, apparently fast asleep. She is strikingly pale.

"She fainted,' Anne explained, "after you introduced her to that boy in the first bed. The sight of the blood transfusion got to her.'

By the time I've carried out a necessarily superficial examination, Sheila is coming around, and is understandably embarrassed.

"I should have told you. The sight of blood always gets to me."

Now it's my turn to be embarrassed. "Oh dear, I should never have put you through this. I've been around here so long I didn't give it a thought."

A few minutes later, after orange juice and a rest in Anne's office chair, Sheila agrees to let her accompany her back to her own department. Despite this early setback, our relationship blossoms, prompting me to explore ending my marriage to Ruth. Ruth has been unwilling to consider it, either because she hopes we might be reunited, or because my monthly child support is way over what the law would require. In April, I take Sheila to England to meet George and Kate, and I take the chance to meet with a divorce lawyer. She assures me I have incontestable grounds for divorce and files for contested divorce hearings. It proves a very formal affair before a woman magistrate in the Inns of Court, with Ruth and I obliged to sit facing each other across a three-foot wide table, while our bewigged and gowned barristers address the magistrate at table's end, largely ignoring us. The settlement proves simple. Ruth must sell our Muswell Hill home and I will receive twelve percent of the sale proceeds. I must pay child support until George and Kate (now twelve and nine) turn eighteen, and I can see them as often as feasible in England or America, with no restrictions.

My solicitor takes Sheila and me out to dinner to celebrate at the One Two One Two restaurant near the Thames Embankment, named for the famous telephone number of its former neighbor, Scotland Yard—Whitehall 1212. The Muswell House sells above the asking price and I duly receive my check. With her share of the proceeds, Ruth buys a three-bedroom house in New Southgate, and Sheila and I are free to marry. But it will be many years before Ruth and I have a conversation that doesn't deteriorate into a shouting match. Even longer before I remember the fun things we did in our fourteen years together, as boyfriend and girlfriend, then husband and wife. And the things I loved about her.

Sheila and I settle on marrying in early November, under the care of my Quaker Gainesville Monthly Meeting at the Thomas Center, the beautiful edifice built in 1906 as a family home—Sunkist Villa—before becoming a hotel where Robert Frost escaped New England's winters. Now Gainesville's Arts and Cultural center, it is a favorite site for weddings. I have been a Quaker ever since Barbara introduced me to them. I had found an instant spiritual home in the silent worship, listening prayerfully for God's "still, small voice," and had more than once valued this deep silence when with a seriously ill or dying child. Our Quaker clerk appoints a "clearness committee" that visits our new home behind Loblolly Woods. Their task is to explore—in a thoroughly Quakerly way—the commitment and constancy of our relationship, and the likelihood of its future success. We must have satisfied them, because next an "oversight committee" is appointed to help us with arrangements for the ceremony. An important item is to find a calligrapher to create the certificate to which all present will "set their hands," and which we will frame and hang on our dining room wall. Back in London, I buy a dress for Kate and a handsome grey suit for George, which I strongly suspect will see only one outing. My sister, Elizabeth, and my eldest nephew come for the November ceremony, and the sun shines as many friends and work colleagues join us in the Turtle Court for the reception. Sheila and I take the overnight plane to London and the following morning board the Orient Express at Waterloo station, bound for Venice. Ten fabulous days' honeymoon in Venice, Florence and Rome, then Sheila announces she's ready for home, itching to get back to a conference deadline, the next draft of a paper, and a teaching course she must prepare for her graduate students.

I'm not sorry to be heading home myself. For the last week, my left eye has been increasingly sore and I've been having trouble tolerating anything more than subdued light. The day after we get home, I find my way to the ophthalmology department and am quickly seated in front of an array of unfamiliar equipment in an exam room. I try to remember when I last sat in a patient's chair other than the dentist's and draw a blank. A man of about fifty with a younger man behind him enters and shakes my hand.

"Bill Driebe. And this is Rob, he's doing a fellowship with us. Don't think we've met. I heard you were having some trouble. How long's it been?"

"Maybe a week, but it's getting worse. I couldn't finish rounds this morning, the light hurt too much."

"Nothing like this before?"

"Nope."

He is dialing back the lumens on his ophthalmoscope, but as soon as he shines the light on my cornea I start to tear up. By the time Rob has taken his turn to look, I can no longer hold my eye open, and he can no longer see beyond my tears.

"Remind you of anything?" Bill quizzes his fellow.

"New to me. Some kind of infection?"

"I don't know what the heck I'm looking at, John" Bill resumes. "Yes, it's an infection, for sure, but it beats me what. Never seen anything quite like it. You wear contacts?"

"Yeah, till last week. Not any more—can't go near them."

My eyes are clamped shut against the glaring overhead lamp.

"Sorry, I'll dim it. Photophobia—people tell me it's hell."

We sit together in shadow. He lays a hand on my arm.

"Your contacts could be the culprit. I'll see you back daily till I nail it. And get Rob hunting down pictures that look like your cornea. Real sorry you're hurting, man. We've got good eye patches, better than Walmart's. And anesthetic drops, along with the antibiotics. I'll get you all you need."

I've never heard a surgeon speak those words. Thirty years a professor and surgeons still fill me with diffidence. Their tight-lipped competence daunts me, how they're thinking and talking on their feet even as they hustle on to their next life-saving task. But Dr. Driebe makes a point of seeing me himself each day, keeping his exams short to minimize my distress, keeping both me and Sheila in the picture about his researching. The diagnosis takes him two weeks: two weeks studying photos in every tome he can lay his hands on, having every ophthalmology faculty member check me out, consulting colleagues across the country. On the fourteenth day, he greets me with the news.

"The eye bank in Atlanta called. They got the answer from the scraping I sent them: *Acanthamoeba* keratitis—it's a parasite, usually found in freshwater lakes, but they've seen a couple of cases linked to contact lens solutions."

He starts me on two eye drops—Baquacil and Brolene, which I have to instill into both eyes every two hours. I've taken sick leave and Sheila is driving me back and forth to the clinic. The drops are some help, but Bill decides the only hope of cure is with a corneal transplant. A week later, more good news.

"Atlanta just called, John—they've got a cornea for you, it'll be here tomorrow. I'm admitting you *stat*, stepping up the drops to hourly."

When I come to sign the consent form, Bill clearly wants to spend time explaining all the possible problems and complications that could arise from the surgery. He even has a couple of articles on corneal transplants for me to read. I surprise myself by wanting to brush them aside.

"Look, Bill, I trust you completely. I know you know what you're doing, and I know you have to put all this stuff in the consent to satisfy the bioethics committee. But just show me where to sign, why don't you!"

When Sheila joins me as I'm being tucked up in bed in a surgical ward, she wants to know chapter and verse of what to expect, and she grabs the articles Bill has handed me, a bit irritated I don't have much to tell her. Only later do I see the irony, given my long time interest in the whole consent process. Perhaps there are others like me, happy to put themselves unconditionally in their caregivers' hands, no questions asked. When I wake through twilight anesthesia some hours later, I reach my arms up through the haze to hug what turns out to be Bill. I grin idiotically at my goof.

"Thought you were Sheila," my voice slurs.

"I talked to her." His face is close to mine, inspecting his handiwork. "She had a whole lot more questions for me than you did! Anyway, no sign of the parasite, man."

I'm back at work two weeks later. I had been certain I would lose the eye, that it would spread to the other one, that I would end up blind, that I would never work again. So now I have been on medicine's receiving end, with a serious, albeit non-fatal, illness, I have a newfound appreciation of what it feels like. And my feelings about surgeons—perhaps deep seated ever since that surgery resident, Dr. W, had yelled across Smithfield market, "Whatever you do, don't take up surgery!"—have softened a whole lot. Thanks, Bill, for your loving care.

Chapter 8: *CREATING*

I take to giving voice to my lifelong love of words—dating back to my early school years—through writing poems. Even with my first raw attempt, penned sitting through a four-hour bioethics meeting, it feels like I've passed into a garden and fallen in love with the resonance of all these beautiful flowers. I'm mostly writing requiems for my young patients, giving voice to whatever surfaced in me during each relationship. The power of scribbling a few lines on a stick-it note quickly catches me up, and I find myself creating oodles of fragments throughout the day's moments, whenever a thought or image, hectic or humdrum, strikes.

I try to capture the final moments of a nineteen-year-old patient I had cared for over the past two years, and watched die by inches over the past two months. Though it may not happen tonight, his nurse, with many years behind her of witnessing these scenarios, has summoned me from home, feeling it could happen any time. I had originally admitted Will as a brawny seventeen-year-old defensive lineman, looking at a scholarship to a Big Ten school—Michigan or Ohio State—with horrendous belly ache and intractable vomiting. A surgical biopsy showed lymphoma that had taken over much of his abdominal cavity. The craggy mass was so matted down on his gut, pancreas and kidneys it was impossible to cut it out without wreaking fatal damage to these organs. With his kidney function worsening hourly, Will, though close to death, responded heroically to our hefty chemotherapy, and a few weeks later a repeat M.R.I. showed the cancer had shrunk to a quarter its original size. But the drugs had inflicted devastating effects on his body, mind and spirit, and the once two-thirty-pound linebacker started resisting our efforts every step of the way.

Looking back, I think he had decided, after those horrendous chemo courses, that he was going to die, and there wasn't one frigging thing this bunch of poison-pushers could do to stop him. It would take four of our stoutest nurses to hold Will down to administer our chemo, and Will's mother, a single woman scarred by an abusive marriage, could do nothing to change his attitude. I tried reasoning, humoring, finally hectoring Will, even calling him a quitter. One of our younger nurses seemed to be making headway—a pretty twenty-two-year-old who was probably getting his testosterone to kick in again. Even in his weakened state, Will reacted to what he read as come-ons by trying to get her between his sheets. I went over every possible approach with my colleagues: Will had a potentially curable cancer, but time was of the essence: if we didn't keep pouring on the chemo, it would take his life in no time flat. Some favored calling in our lawyers, arguing he was incompetent to make rational decisions in his current state. But I reminded them that, unless we could prove definitively that Will was mentally impaired, we could not, legally or ethically, challenge his decision to refuse more treatment, even if we thought it could cure him.

But this one-hundred-million dollar question—was Will of sufficient maturity and intelligence, and in sound enough mind, to make this decision on his own behalf?—was moot. How did any of us think we were going to do battle with this Randy White of a defensive tackle? He might be down but he would fight us to the end. If he was to die, let it be with a mite of dignity. His mother started siding with her son, even if more from intimidation than anything else. My colleagues finally conceded: don't call in the lawyers, even an ethics committee. Just give Will as much comfort and dignity as possible. Hence my poem, prompted by his refusing my help as he strained to lift his cup. Earlier, he'd surrendered and let his mom and the nurses bathe him like a baby, but he still struggled to shave himself. I had witnessed the shrinking to nothingness in a few weeks of those potent deltoids, triceps, biceps. All my instincts rebelled, but I held my peace, sat close to his bed, tuned into his stertorous breathing, and prayed his transition would be quick and peaceful.

The start and end of my poem to Will:

I yearn to shout for you, dear ill one, for
the waste of muscle wraps that droop upon
the once potent bones of youth. . . .

I want to howl,
once wild one, swathed in your bleak crib

whence the catheter dangles: Why do you
rail no more against your closing curfew?

Another child's mother called me at four-thirty one morning. She was mad, and she was scared. Mad because I hadn't figured out what was happening to Ben; scared for the exact same reason. I had been caring for her twelve-year-old since he developed a brain tumor earlier in the year. After a raft of chemo, he had received a stem cell transplant two weeks earlier, then in the late evening suffered an epileptic seizure out of the blue. It had lasted an hour—a life time both for Mom and us—and took massive doses of anti-seizure meds to arrest it. He was running a fever of 104°—something else I had no explanation for. Blood and urine cultures, a lumbar puncture to rule out meningitis, a C.A.T. scan to look for a brain abscess—drew a blank. Good news so far as it goes, but no help in dredging up answers to Mom's frantic questions. Once Ben was settled into deep sleep, and I was sure he had enough medication on board to forestall further fits, I did what I could to reassure Mom:

"Things really do seem under control. I don't think anything more will happen tonight. It's not so unusual at times like this to not have all the answers. Can you try to put your mind at rest, maybe catch some sleep? The nurses will call me right away for anything else."

I had headed home to catch a few more hours sleep before daylight. Meanwhile, Mom spent these hours perched at her son's unconscious body, questions swirling about in her mind:

What's happening? Is he going to make it? What can I do to help?

Finally, she had to unleash her pent-up questions on someone, and I was the obvious target. She was mad that I could take off home to bed when she was sure her son would die any minute. Hence the second call in the early hours, her outburst leaping over me down the telephone line. During our thirty-minute call, we ran the gamut of human emotions, not least because her voice had triggered long-buried memories within me. My subsequent poem tried to capture the images flashing back to Uncle Ken's rages at my fourteen-year-old self, while I fought off exhaustion. Mom left me no moment to respond, so I listened mutely to her outpouring. Then over several agonizing minutes, her voice quieted and slowed, the storm finally spent, allowing me a far more comforting image—that of own mom comforting me after waking from a nightmare. Ben's mother at last stopped long enough to absorb my cautious words of hope, even let herself laugh a little—at me? at herself? at the whole mystifying passage of events?—and ended up offering me her support. Here are sections from my poem, "Fear," reflecting on this episode:

> *Four-thirty on my phone.*
> *A hard hail of fear hits me, icing the voice . . .*
> *Why's he getting worse?*
> *When will his fever break?*
> *Will the seizures come again?*
> *. . . unraveling a flash of Uncle's angry eyes pounding*
> *down on my adolescent energy . . .*
> *then amidst the tumult I hear the soothe*
> *of my mother's murmuring . . .*
> *my mind retakes its presence here,*
> *hears at last this mother hearing me . . .*
> *It's working, isn't it? You know, don't you?*
> *Don't change things. Glad we talked: thanks.*

Poetry is helping me realize the richness of the loving relationships in my work, across age, sex, ethnicity, education. Bringing down the artificial barriers society erects between us. It is restoring, *re-storying*, me by bringing me back to my center, at times my mind and spirit feel scattered to the winds. I am giving vocal expression to my deepest feelings, reclaiming my authentic self, sorting out deep-seated confusions within me. Poems are risky; you can't duck their truth. In sorting reality from illusion, they take no prisoners. But their words are allies, challenging and strengthening me with their fidelity and beauty. Drawing on my work with these children, families, and co-workers, reflecting the rhythm arising from the polarities and synergies of our lives, they move from inexplicable to explicable, from dark to light.

A phone call at home one Sunday morning: "John?"
"Hello."
"Mary Lane, Tim Lane's wife—head of Orthopedics at North Florida Regional. I read your article about using art in the hospital. Can we meet?"
I carry the phone onto our patio, bathed in the early sun. "Great—you're my first feedback."

"I want to talk some more about your ideas. I'm both a nurse and a painter, and I think you're onto something important."

The local physicians' magazine had published my article, "Art in Medicine: Exploring the Connection," about a half-day symposium I had run the month before at the health center. I was raising a question pushing its way into my consciousness: Could we add a prescription of *art* to all our cutting-edge medicine, with its exclusive focus on science and technology? My prime mover was poet John Keats, who in 1817 wrote, one year after graduating from Guy's Hospital: "I am certain of nothing but the holiness of the heart's affection, and the truth of the imagination." Then I had come on those of fellow pediatrician and renowned poet, William Carlos Williams: "It is difficult to get the news from poems, but men die miserably every day for lack of what is found there." My third light bulb had been a more immediate *Aha!* moment: my child patients always seemed to turn to art-making to rescue meaning and harmony from the chaos of current catastrophe, knowing instinctively the power of paint and song and dance to come to their aid.

So why not grown-ups, too? For my symposium, I invited a four-piece physician band, The Docs of Dixie, plus a local painter, a poet, and an actor from University of Florida's Arts Department to first perform for our audience, then talk about how they saw art as nourishing their minds and bodies. About a hundred people showed up, so I was clearly speaking to something dormant in many coworkers. But I had had no further reaction to either symposium or article—until now. Mary and I decided to meet next afternoon for tea at a local bistro, quickly moving on to wine as we brainstormed ideas back and forth.

"I know every artist in town," Mary exclaims. "Why don't we have a gathering at my home, then talk it up with the hospital nurses. We could do some Atrium performances, then move on up to the wards. Bring musicians, painters, poets, right to the patients' bedsides!"

"Hey, why not? They'll have a hard time firing a tenured prof—even if this isn't in my job description."

"I love it!" Mary is jumping up and down, and I have to grab her wine glass as it threatens to tumble off the table. "This is brilliant! Let's do it!"

The call for artists is a sellout. Twenty-two painters, poets, musicians, storytellers, sculptors and dancers gather around our common intent: *heal our hospital with art!* No one queries if art is good for whatever ails you. We decide to start on the stem cell transplant unit—a risky first choice. Bringing artists unversed in hospital rules into this ultra-sterile intensive care unit, filled with many of the hospital's sickest patients, is surely pushing the envelope. But Mary cuts through my misgivings.

"Come on, you're in charge up there, John. So where better?"

"Well, those patients could certainly use some fun—probably more than anyone."

We bring four artists to meet the nurses, and questions immediately surface. Can we launch this grassroots movement without the okay of the powers-that-be? Can we pay the artists for their time and talent? Do we need written protocols? How do we tell if we're doing any good? What advocates do we need to open doors and troubleshoot problems?

"So who are your first artists?" Helen, the unit's nurse manager, asks Mary, when we go over details of our proposal.

"My friend, Mary Lisa. She's got art supplies up the gazoo—coloring stuff, modeling clay. Drums even. And we'll have our guitarist, Jerry, serenading patients and nurses, both!"

We christen ourselves Arts in Medicine—*aka* AIM—and hold journaling, drumming, and T-shirt-painting workshops. We introduce weekly music and dance sessions for the unit's patients sitting masked and gowned in the corridor outside their isolation rooms. They take pride in their creative accomplishments, and seem happier and better adjusted to the ordeals they must endure. The nurses, meanwhile, are getting to know them and each other on a whole new level. Morale is at an all-time high.

We run into obstacles. The unpaid time artists can offer is limited, and at first the intensive-care atmosphere scares them. We have to raise the thorny question of "professional" clothing and behavior with a few of our musicians. But as word spreads, and we move to other hospital units, we begin gathering artist stories and feedback from patients, families, and staff. We are unsure how we will use this as evidence of benefit—it hardly lends itself to the carefully constructed clinical trials I'm so used to. We may already be convinced that art-making is good for whatever ails your body, mind or spirit, but helping others to see this truth and embrace it in their daily lives will be a trick. Our best evaluations are the wonderful quotes from patients we collect: "I was just happy to see someone walk in without needles;" "Fear can be a killer—give us more art;" "A wonderful help during long waits in the hospital;" "It helps us share our uniqueness;" "In the midst of illness, I found art again;" "Getting transfusions sucks, but I have fun knowing how to make stuff;" "Thank you, thank you, and God bless you all." And from the mom of a very sick child: "He painted his view of earth from heaven." And the comments from the hospital staff and students: "Could we get this course every week?" "AIM should be mandatory for us all;" "Art creates a humane environment for patients and families;" "I felt childlike feelings . . . more human doing this;" "Thank you for beautifying our hospital, and giving our patients new life;" "Self-expression is especially important when you're overwhelmed by crisis;" "Enriches the lives of patients and staff on the front lines;" "I was brought to deep communion;" "The smiles on those kids' faces made my day."

On a chilly Thursday morning seven days before Christmas, eight of us gather in a small windowless conference room to celebrate both the season and the six-month anniversary of Arts in Medicine. We are taking time in this cozy space, normally set aside as a quiet room for grieving families, to wrap a layer of safety about us as we listen to each other. As the stories flow—poignant patient vignettes, personal life challenges—I reflect how far removed I am from the S.O.A.P. (Subjective, Objective, Assessment, Plan) notes American resident doctors use to report on their patients to their attending physicians.

Jane tells of Mrs. Partridge, dying with leukemia on ward 7B. She is ninety-two, wears a pink chiffon nightdress with matching hair ribbon. Once a New York model, she had seen Isadora Duncan dance, so Jane and Claire had performed dances from "Cherubim," "Narcissus," and "Blessed Spirits" right there in the ward, with Mrs. Partridge joining in. Mary-Lisa tells of Harriet, a twenty-two-year-old woman facing a bleak outlook. Harriet loves the beach, so Mary-Lisa had decorated a long silk scarf with seagulls and shells and draped it across her bed. Ellie speaks of the poem she had created with Labron, a fourteen-year-old recovering from a painful sickle cell crisis. Their subject is friendship: they have composed alternate lines, with Labron helping Gabrielle set it to music, and printing a copy for him to share with his classmates. Then it's my turn to talk about Storytelling Hour in "Charlie's Corner," the oncology unit's family room, that Thanksgiving weekend.

"Our mostly middle-aged patients trail their I.V. poles towards the armchairs, while luckier families are sharing feasts at firesides or on their decks. Don, the hospice chaplain, leads off with a childhood memory of sugar-cane farming. His uncle had always let the mule have a good long slurp of cane syrup before hauling the tractor off to the boiling vats. Bob, a hard-scrabble Florida boy, talks about getting sick and having to listen from his bed to the happy voices at the groaning Thanksgiving tables below his window. Liza tells of her toddler sister wedging a fragment of chicken up her nose that wasn't sniffed out for a week.

"Cancer and chemo are forgotten as Charlie's Corner takes on its holiday-time reality. Finally, Don evokes the Thanksgiving spirit by recalling how the Mayflower's pilgrims had offered prayers of thanks, despite half of them having died that first terrible year. Time to serenade the nurses—after all, they are stuck in hospital for the holiday, too. All the favorites are trotted out, after a reminder that harmonizing is 'just singing any note no one else is singing!' The ragged voices of five patients and five volunteers carry through the ward, amidst laughter, tears, and thanksgiving by all. As these caregivers become the recipients of loving care from the very people they are here to serve, the shared stories and off-note singing have taken us all a few steps further along our healing journeys."

Jill, our dancer, tells the remarkable story of fifteen-year-old Brandisha. "She's back in with another sickle pain crisis. Just like bad frostbite, but in back and legs and stomach all at once. Her red cells get bent out of shape during cold weather or an infection and dam up her blood vessels. The residents just hook her up to morphine round-the-clock every time she gets admitted, and it can take a week for the crisis to pass. But this time something miraculous happens. When I visit her, she looks zonked out with narcotic, but she's got her ear buds in and is rolling her whole body rhythmically side-to-side on her pillows. It turns out she's listening to Beethoven's *Pastoral*—not at all what I'd expected.

"'Is this what you usually listen to?' I quiz her.

"'Yeah.'

"A light bulb goes off—swinging to Beethoven: why not?

"'You like to dance, Brandisha?'

"She grins, humoring me. I've brought my multicolored silk scarves, so I start sweeping them back and forth in a soothing rhythm. Suddenly, her hospital room transforms into a unique performance stage. Brandisha follows the flow with her body, hips moving rhythmically below the bed covers. Then I help her to her feet and we dance in unison all around her bed, arms swinging the scarves and tumbling together like waves, Brandisha smiling dreamily all the while.

"'How is it?' I quiz her.

"'Real nice.'

"'Does it help your pain?'"
"'Yeah. Doesn't bother me anymore.'"

Our conference room is silent, rapt in Jill's story, tears gathering under many eyelids. I have admitted Brandisha myself many times and always ordered up the same old high-dose I.V. opioid. Now here she is, tapping into her own supply of internal pain-banishing morphine. I break the silence.

"So has Amos" (my on-duty colleague) "backed off her morphine?"

"Right! Brandisha wanted to stop it altogether, says she much prefers music and dancing because it doesn't leave her zonked out. So he cut it by fifty percent, and her pain is down from a *ten* to a *two*!"

"She *has* to be releasing her own endorphins. You know what Salvador Dali said—'I don't do drugs, I *am* drugs.'"

"That has to be it, John," Jill agrees. "I've been reading about how pain can trigger your own narcotic. Like a runner's high, or maybe deep meditation—you get right in the zone." She looks around at the other artists. "You know, it happened to me when I first started dancing as a teenager. I would become utterly relaxed but energized at the same time. The psychologists are calling it '*flow*'—being so intensely immersed everything else disappears."

"A real coincidence," I add. "Sheila and I were at the American Psychological Association conference last fall, and we heard a keynote from Mike Csikszentmihalyi—the guru of flow states. We've just had a wonderful live demo of his theory."

In the New Year, Mary and I find ourselves at the hospital C.E.O.'s monthly administration conference to present our findings after A.I.M.'s first year. Paul Metts sits at the end of the long polished table, his numerous V.P.'s arrayed down the sides. Mary and I take the vacant seats by the double doors and proceed with our slides. We show a storyteller at a patient's bedside, a poet and dancer doing a presentation in the hospital atrium, a group of medical students writing poetry, the state governor and his wife painting six-inch ceramic tiles for a collage to grace the hospital walls. We have charted a breakdown of one-thousand surveys of the responses from patients, families and staff to A.I.M.'s presence and performances, turning them into pretty compelling stats about the many benefits to bodies, minds, and spirits of our participants. Paul glances down the table.

"Comments, anyone?"

A few nods, and a number of complementary words. He addresses me. "So what d'you want from us?"

I summon up my quite unrehearsed response: "$50,000 for the next year—to pay eight part-time artists. Plus supplies of course."

Another brief survey down the table: "I think we can manage that. To be reviewed at the end of a year's trial, of course."

With swift words of thanks, Mary and I are out the door before they can change their minds. Five days later, A.I.M. finds itself the proud owner of a new budget line administered by the Patient Care and Public Relations department, soon to become a permanent item on the multimillion-dollar Shands budget.

A few months later, Mary and I write up this first year's activities to publish in a nursing journal. We have discovered we're not alone in embarking on similar enterprises, so there has to be a readership out there. I decide to include the story of Brenda, blessed with three beautiful children, with a successful realty business—and with aplastic anemia. For no good reason, her bone marrow has gone totally on the blink, leaving her abruptly short of the red and white blood cells and platelets so vital to her survival. She had become exhausted, menorrhagic from being unable to clot her blood, and defenseless against any known bug.

"I get up one morning, and find myself in an alien country where no one speaks my language," is how Brenda describes it. "And I have to put myself in the hands of all these total strangers."

She has joined the ranks of those who are assaulted by sudden, inexplicable illness. But once the initial horrors of blood and bone marrow tests, I.V. antibiotics, and blood and platelet transfusions have slowed, Brenda takes some solace in knowing what she is up against: a stem cell transplant to give her a brand new bone marrow and hopefully cure her. Stuck in one of our unit's isolation rooms with a lot of time on her hands, she daydreams about how to make the best of her day.

"I wake one morning from a dream of myself as a little girl making pictures. Which is about the age I'm feeling right now in real life—a new six-year-old kid on the block."

Mary Lisa shows up and Brenda tentatively enquires about art supplies. Within minutes, she finds herself possessed of liquid paints and a sketch pad and starts creating nameless multicolors of swirls and shapes and blotches.

"My pictures become my new best friends. I can run away and hide in them, tell them everything I'm thinking and feeling, and they never answer back. When I'm fretting about my children and husband, wondering how they're coping without me, some part of me reasserts itself. Like I'm praying, letting go and letting God, as the Quakers say. Who'd have thunk it?"

"You're a courageous woman, Brenda," Mary Lisa tells her. "Here you are, ripped from your day-to-day life in the scariest way, and you're coping with just a couple of paint brushes for company. You don't need me, just my art supplies!"

Mary and I talk with another artist, Tina Mullen, who has created an art gallery outside the Cancer Centre with the money put up by several physicians. We decide to beautify the walls of the hospital atrium, not just with pictures but with ceramic tile collages made by patients and families. Over the next several months, we accumulate more than a thousand of these four-by-four-inch tiles, and Lee Anne, another artist, takes on the task of firing them and constructing two "healing walls." We stage a formal opening ceremony, with hundreds attending. For the countless patients, staff and students who hurry through the atrium, or linger to chat at the coffee stand, this wall-length installation is an arresting sight. We ask people at random to tell us what they see.

"The tiles are like a welcome;" "I get a chance to stop and rest a minute;" "They help me find my way;" "Maybe I don't need my doctor's appointment after all!"

Then Mary Lisa hits on a new-but-old concept. "What about all our patients? They spend hours every day just staring at the ceiling. Well, those plasterboard tiles on their ceilings will take tempura paint beautifully. And they're only twelve inches by twelve—perfect for a canvas! Why not give the patients something fun to look at, too?"

None of us have heard of decorating ceilings, at least not since Michelangelo painted the ceiling of the Sistine Chapel in the Apostolic Palace.

"That's a brilliant idea. After all, very few patients get to see our atrium displays. But I don't think we can just start taking the ceiling tiles down ourselves. You've been around this place a while now, have you got to know any of the maintenance guys?"

Mary Lisa grins. "As a matter of fact, I have. So has Tina. I just bet they'd be willing to take a few down and replace them in their spare time! And of course we won't need to do the painting. We've got a zillion Brendas for that," she adds, which gets us all laughing.

Our maintenance staff gets into the spirit of this new venture, and if we thought "Healing Ceilings" would stay confined to the stem cell transplant or the pediatric unit, we were way wrong. Geriatrics soon wants in on the action, and other wards and outpatient clinics start vying for the brightest and most decorative ceilings in the hospital. Before long, there are painted ceilings in hospital units and clinics everywhere. Then the medical and nursing students start putting plasterboard tiles up on their classroom ceilings. The whole hospital takes on the look of a unique art gallery.

I run into a Professor of English and Theatre, Sid Homan, a lifetime story teller who agrees to start telling his tales to our patients. He begins on our transplant unit, then expands to the psychiatric ward, where he adds theatre games to help teenagers with their crucial need to express their feelings.

"I tell a lot of stories about kids I knew growing up in South Philadelphia. It doesn't get much rougher than that," Sid tells me. "So I see the teens and younger adults using my stories as mirrors of their own lives, from their carefree childhoods to their current conflicts."

The program is so successful that six months later Sid hands me a pre-print of "A Fish in the Moonlight," the book he's about to publish of these experiences. I place it in a binder in Charlie's Corner and several other patient and family rooms. Then I remember what he had told me about actors doing pre-performance warm-ups, how the theatre can teach us about working with patients and families. I ask Sid if he would talk to our medical students. He starts with small groups, using role play to help them get comfy in the scenarios they will undoubtedly encounter.

"Developing an actor's awareness doesn't lessen the reality," he tells them. "It's like watching yourself on video, you can rehearse beforehand. Now who's going to be the doctor and who the patient?" Two of the students reluctantly volunteer. "Now imagine you have to give some difficult tidings to your patient," he tells the doctor-actor. "You're going to open the door, walk across the room, greet the patient, sit down, and announce your news." He turns to the other student. "Now, I need you as patient to react appropriately, make it realistic. Don't worry, guys, there's no one else here, just the three of us."

The other half-dozen students guffaw, perhaps from discomfort in this new situation. Sid has them all try out various options.

"Just how do you open the door? Firmly, with confidence? Or tentatively, so as not to alarm the patient? What signals do you give, if any? How quickly do you cross the room to greet your patient? When do you sit, and how close? How do you phrase your information? Do you get right to the point, or do you approach it gradually? Do you touch the patient? How long do you wait? And just how do you exit?"

Each actor-student responds differently. They turn out to be more comfy in their patient roles, and even help their "doctor" classmates adapt their performance to make them more genuine and compassionate.

"This stuff doesn't come at all naturally," one says. "It's like being engaged and disengaged at the same time. I guess it takes a lot of practice to get good at it."

I reflect on how helpful this could be if it were in the medical school curriculum. I certainly had no mentors telling me about any of this, so I had to learn the hard way. But my experience as an actor on stage certainly helped me.

Mary and I start hearing more and more about arts programs in other medical centers around the country. It seems like a grassroots movement has sprung up among like-spirited souls who share our vision, without any systematic planning or communication between us. We give a presentation about A.I.M. at a national conference of the newly formed Society for Arts in Healthcare in San Francisco. A far cry from the cancer and transplant conferences I'm so used to, awash with oncologists and scientists fighting for the competitive edge. At the registration desk, artists of every stripe mingle with nurses, child life workers, even a few doctors and patients. Our own session attracts a big crowd, with nobody from the audience wanting to grandstand and present their own data during question time. The energy at the nightly performances and keynotes is so charged no one wants to go to bed.

We decide to host our own arts and healing symposium, and a committee meets together for a year, led by our visionary writer-in-residence, Gail Ellison. "Restorying Lives, Restoring Selves" draws two-hundred-plus friends and allies together at Shands and our local art museum. We stage fifty presentations, ranging from acrobats and actors to clowns and curators, from dancers and designers to gourmet cooks and gerontologists, from painters and poets to psychologists and story tellers, from rock musicians to yoga instructors. Our keynoters are Annette Ridenour, president of Aesthetics, on designing hospital way-finding, Gina Halpern, curator of the Body & Soul exhibit, on visual art and health; Kim Tanzer, from our College of Architecture, on holistic architecture; and Michael Samuels, who directs Art as a Healing Force, on imagery in cancer therapy. Stuart Pimsler and Suzanne Costello, co-directors of the Ohio Dance Company, present a communal dance called "Caring for the Caregiver," and not a soul is excluded as we dance in joyful assembly into the evening hours, with a scattering of wheelchairs leading the light fantastic. Last, but by no means least, comes six-foot-six Dr. Patch Adams, founder of the Gesundheit Institute, on "Humor and Health: Rationale for a Clown's Life."

Patch had arrived the afternoon before, and somehow found his way to my clinic as I was checking on the children still receiving their chemo infusions. I had just finished fixing a little guy's I.V. site when I found myself swept up into Patch's arms, and the whole clinic—patients, parents, nurses—erupted in laughter as we proceeded to complete rounds together with me hoisted aloft. Afterwards, Patch and I had supper together at a downtown restaurant.

"John, I'm leading another clown mission to Russia in November. I want you to join us, then come and work with me in West Virginia. We're building our free community hospital in an ecovillage—a health center based on friendship and creativity, and a whole lot of goofiness! The pay's not much, but you'll be among your own kind—I can always spot a natural clown!"

After a second beer, I start feeling tempted. The idea of travelling the world with Patch's clown team, bringing exuberant healing energy to people the world over is enormously appealing. "I can be very seductive, John," Patch murmurs, not for the first time. "I promise you you'll never have another bad day!" After the symposium, we are joined by Sheila. She and I had talked long into the previous evening, and she had caught the excitement I was feeling. But as the three of us go back and forth over the pros and cons of what Patch proposes, tension builds between my charismatic new medical colleague and my new wife. I finally have to acknowledge it: Sheila is the only one of us with her feet planted firmly on the ground. She hasn't actually come out and said it, but I know the life Patch proposes would never be for her, and I know instantly where my loyalties lie.

"Patch, you're dead right, you *are* very seductive. And you're right, our medical system is deeply flawed. But if I'm to be an activist, it has to be from *within* this system—warts and all."

But his courageous and crazy convictions stay with me. Why indeed can't loving kindness and compassion, and a whole lot of laughter and joy, claim their central place in our caregiving? I may not be ready to rebel against our teaching hospital's dress code, and adopt a complete clown outfit, but I can certainly push the envelope. We doctors are obliged to wear ties, so I acquire a holey "Swiss cheese" one, made entirely of expandable elastic, complete with a nibbling mouse hanging off its end. I take to wearing colorful odd socks, which quickly become a trademark with my patients, and carry in my pockets an array of squeaky toys, clown masks and wigs, red noses, and a three-foot-square Union Jack handkerchief. I quickly find grown-ups enjoy an impromptu clown display just as much when the moment seems to call for it.

My three-foot-square handkerchief can bring some healing humor to hard situations. I had just broken the news to a teenaged patient, Jess, and his parents that he would have to receive several more rounds of chemo for his cancer—something none of them had prepared for. Mom starts to cry, and both Jess and his dad do their awkward best to comfort her. After a few minutes, Mom starts to dry her eyes and tries for a small grin. Which turns to a much larger one on all sides when I take a very long drawn-out moment to haul my Union Jack hankie out of my pants pocket and offer it to her.

Then a new patient gives me a powerful reminder of humor's healing power. When I had first met Leah, she had already received her first chemo doses for her bone cancer, leaving her mouth and throat raw and painful. A debilitating side effect almost impossible to prevent, or even relieve. That, coupled with the pain caused by the large mass in her iliac crest, had put her in a thoroughly grumpy mood that Monday morning towards the whole medical profession. And as I was to find out, Leah didn't hesitate to make her feelings known. As I approach her bedside to introduce myself, she reaches up, grabs my tie, and yanks it hard. I instantly regret I'm not wearing my expandable rubber one.

"Give me morphine," she croaks through cracked lips.

A quick check reveals the horrid inflammation and ulceration of the lining of her mouth and throat, and I write for a stat dose of narcotic to ease her pain. Twenty-four hours on, I'm at her bedside once more—this time making sure I am wearing my cheese tie. She presents me with a cartoon drawing of the two of us, capturing Leah's own very real anger and her new doctor's astonishment at being greeted with physical assault. The time intervening between my two visits has been long enough for my feisty patient to reassert her sense of humor, and to put artistry to work to capture the moment of our first meeting. Once she's fully recovered, Leah comes to see me in my office, and I bemoan the fact I have changed offices half a dozen times during my tenure, never once meriting a window. Three days later, she reappears with a beautiful two-by-three foot image of a stained-glass window to grace the wall in front of my desk. No depiction of a religious icon, though—it's a lifelike rendition of Kermit and Miss Piggy, hand-in-hand and gazing soulfully into each other's eyes.

Some months on, Leah goes on to receive an autologous transplant to try to completely eradicate her sarcoma, but tragically the cancer recurs in hip and lungs. Meanwhile, she finds the energy to work on a thirty-four page coloring book for young patients going through such therapies. Each image shows a cartoon self-portrait of a much younger Leah, capturing the whole experience a child can expect, all drawn in broad outlines to leave space for coloring. In the first frame, a nurse is checking her vital signs as Leah clutches her teddy bear; then another nurse is drawing a blood sample from her infusaport; she depicts herself sitting in front of a massive machine for whole-body irradiation; then curled up in bed while envisioning a favorite place she will visit once she's out of here. The final portrait shows a six-year-old Leah leaving the hospital hand-in-hand with Dad. No surprise to learn that Leah has earned a full scholarship to the University of Chicago to study for her M.F.A. in Fine Arts, even though we both know it is unlikely she will even start her graduate work this coming fall. Somewhere along the line, she links up with boyfriend Josh, and towards the end of her long battle with cancer they appear in my office to announce that they are getting married. By this time, Leah has taken to making clinic visits without her parents.

"They always ask to come, doc—only cave when I promise I'll report back to them in full. The thing is, I can take whatever you dish out, about, when it's just Josh and me. But when Mom loses it, I start in too. Then Dad, he gets to disputing every word you say. Too much, I just stop thinking."

"I get the picture, Leah."

As she shifts her weight from one side to the other, I can see she is sparing her left hip, the site of the cancer's greatest concentration.

"So I want the straight poop—none of that flapdoodle you dish out to my folks, okay?"

This at a time when the straight poop is that her cancer is fast getting the better of her. And today my clinic happens to be especially congested. I had known it was going to be that way when I'd tried to slip through the waiting area many hours earlier, only to be importuned by two "problem parents" before I had made it to the nurses' station.

"You know me, aren't I always the up-front shooter, Leah?"

But it isn't easy telling the unvarnished truth to anyone, however courageous and forthright they may be, when that truth is she has only a short time left on this earth. The radiologist had called me within a half-hour of Leah completing her latest X-rays: never a good sign—X-ray reports are usually on a twenty-four-hour turn-around. The cancer has spread to both shoulders and her backbone. Not for the first time, I had found myself wondering why I hadn't become a radiologist: the ultimate desk job, sitting at the X-ray screen dishing out life-and-death judgments to those on the front line, leaving us to come up with the words that will turn their terse reports into something a patient can hear and make sense of.

Leah's reaction to my news of how far the cancer has spread is the wry comment: "It's not dying I mind so much, doc—but just not in diapers, okay?" She throws a look at Josh, who summons a sheepish grin, even though he is as near tearing up as I am. "Well, babe, I just hope you find another girl as good as me. Even if my body is in its urn, I'll be watching you so you'd better treat her right! Right now, though, we're going to set up house, you and me. Wedding pictures on the mantle, you bringing me breakfast in bed, all that stuff married people do."

I have no answer to her courageous levity, just a big lump in my throat.

"So you don't want to turn me into a guinea pig?"

She is referring to the many discussions we have had about more experimental drugs we can try. I know very well her jaundiced view of *that* course of action.

"Well, there's always another drug around the corner, Leah—but I'd be fooling both of us if I claimed it would make any long term difference."

"So—how long have I got?"

That's always the question—the one with no pat answer. The way her cancer is spreading she could be dead in a week. But Leah is a fighter, and if she has some things she wants to get done she could be around for months.

"How long do *you* think?"

"Hey, you're the doc, you tell me!"

"Well, I wasn't exactly joking, Leah. Folks like you have a lot to say about how long—along with God, of course."

"Josh wants us to honeymoon at Disney—so don't hold back on the morphine. I want to be able to make those rides."

They did indeed get married, and did get to spend their weekend honeymoon at Disneyworld. By that time, Leah was in the inevitable diapers, with Josh changing them as need be. I wrote this requiem, *Breaking News*, to celebrate Leah's life and her brave death. This is a fragment from my poem:

> *In the cancer clinic, people brush us as we seek*
> *the sanctuary of an empty room to visit death together.*
> *Leah, dying's fine, I say (to myself: what do I know?)*
> *as you, knowing death too well, assuage me. You fear*
> *not dying but doing it (who wouldn't?) in diapers.*
> *You're shy telling Josh: I still, presumptuously, love you;*
> *in time you'll ride, in morphine-trails, your last carousel.*

I come across a quote by fellow physician Ernst Wynder: "The function of medicine is to have people die young as late as possible." Which sets me looking for what else is out there, and I quickly uncover evidence that simply playing together can offer measurable benefit to the health of our bodies, minds, and spirits. Norman Cousins started what has become a movement when he was diagnosed with ankylosing spondylitis back in 1979, and found he could get prolonged spells of pain-free sleep after ten minutes of belly laughter. He called it "internal jogging." By a happy stroke of serendipity, I run into an occupational therapist and a recreational therapist who are exploring how to use humor in the psychiatric unit they work in. My new friends, Mary and Jane, and I decide our hospital is long overdue for a little lightening up, so we start offering "laughter and playshops" to nurses and medical technicians, social workers and dieticians, even the hospital accounting office, as a new A.I.M. venture. The question we pose to ourselves and our fast-growing groups of participants comes down to: "Can work and fun coexist in the same sentence?"

Our timing is good, because the hospital is undergoing a major cost-cutting overhaul, with dozens of staff layoffs, morale slumping, tensions rising, and scapegoats being sought on all sides. My senior nursing friend,

Helen, suggests we might raise the mood of the end-of-year staff meeting—though she mutters beforehand, "It'll be hard going, John, things are at an all time low." With this counsel ringing in our ears, and decked out in clown gear and carting toys, funny noses and balloons, we arrive to strut our stuff in front of seventy-five "survivors" of the latest round of layoffs. Off we go with our opener—free-for-all bubble blowing and marshmallow fights—followed by our "cow, duck, pig" mixer ("Find your own herd, flock, or sty by honk-moo-quacking the appropriate noise"). Within minutes, there is total uproar as a tidal wave of pent-up feelings spill forth and people start falling about like five-year-olds. I catch sight of the hospital CEO and the VP for Nursing dancing back-to-back, as others line up for the chance to scream incoherently while jumping up and down on our rubber "tantrum mats."

We finally get everyone settled down enough to stretch out on the floor for story time, and leave in the knowledge that the research is right: laughter can be a healing force, and we had seen some real healing of wounds here. As artist-philosopher Elbert Hubbard put it, "Don't take life too seriously, or you won't get out alive."

Our growing belief in the healing power of art inspires Jill, Rusti Brandman from the university's Dance faculty and me to build on A.I.M.'s strictly patient-centered focus. We decide to create a Center for Arts Medicine in the College of Art, focusing on teaching and research. The Dean is hugely supportive, and we gather interest and sponsorship around the university and beyond. We create a second website (www.arts.ufl.edu/cam) to distinguish this new university-wide initiative from our hospital-based A.I.M. (www.artsinmedicine.ufhealth.org) which is strictly patient-focused. Our new Center will teach undergraduate and graduate courses, as well as hosting an annual summer intensive to attract people from around the nation.

I feel more and more like an artist cut loose in medical science's domain. As if I've been slipping in sideways all along my love for the multimedia duet of song and dance and play. Never again will I let information technology—that endless round of automated blood tests and diagnostic biopsies, of C.T. and M.R.I. and P.E.T. scans, all assigned to remote electronic records—come between me and the richness, intimacy, and innate intelligence of my patients' stories. Our indigenous peoples the world over have always known art's sacred power to heal. What a "for-people-not-profit" synergy there is in this, in art as science's companion as a balm for our bodies, our minds, and our spirits. I am invited to present A.I.M. at the annual conference of the American Holistic Medical Association. It has been two years since I attended a physician conference other than our national oncology gatherings—and I'm not missing it one bit.

I had never heard of this group before, but a glance at their website tells me its goal is "to transform conventional healthcare into a more holistic model, creating a safe harbor for physician pioneers, and for students of integrative and holistic medicine." I like that word, *holistic*—it is how I describe what I am teaching in the elective course I've inserted into our medical school's curriculum. I had entitled an article of mine "Teaching Holistic Medicine is Not the Same as Teaching C.A.M." [C.A.M. is a shortening for complementary & alternative medicine—the widely accepted term to cover the upsurge of public interest in treatments outside accepted "evidence-based" medicine.] I have christened my course "Holism,101," defining holistic medicine as the art and science of healing the whole person in relation to every person's community and environment. I limit the sign-up to six, and we start off the month by sitting around my office floor telling stories. I encourage talking about patients they have known, because this is the easiest place to get them started—and it's really what they want to talk about. These are all fourth-year students who have spent the past three years presenting their rushed and stylized S.O.A.P. patient notes to their attendings on early morning rounds. Now they have the chance to reflect on some they especially recall, after caring for them often for quite brief periods of time.

As we cozy up on the floor of my eight-by-eight-foot office, the stories that flow forth are just like the ones at our Thursday morning A.I.M. rounds, entirely concerned with the *subjective*: not just about the patient's story, but the relationship that has grown between giver and receiver of care. We reflect on the two-way nature of this relationship, that arises from being respected and trusted, and almost always liked. Something that builds these students' resilience, autonomy, self-confidence, as they develop into professional caregivers. I think back to my own med school days, how I lacked any kind of guidance of this kind. Our medical curriculum has certainly come along way. Jeff recalls a seventy-two-year-old German immigrant, who is a heart transplant survivor, and tells his story through Hans' own voice, reading from the journal he had kept intermittently during school.

"I made it through the firebombing at the end of World War II, but

I've never forgotten it. A bomb exploded over our heads, and we were trying to get out of the building when the roof caught fire. After that, I reckoned I could deal with about anything. Before I got my heart transplant, I had one foot in the grave, but someone had to die for me to live. They're in short supply, too—I have no idea how they decide who gets the next one."

Hans makes many trips in for check-ups, Jeff tells us, and has to swallow a boatload of medicines to prevent rejection of his donated heart and other problems. "I've always been a sociable guy, and I got to know a lot of the regulars. So I organized get-togethers while we were waiting on our check-ups—there could be ten of us. At first, it was all talk about our illnesses and surgeries and stuff, but then we'd start chatting about our families, and sometimes share our childhood memories. I could have written half a dozen books with all those stories."

Jeff had encouraged Hans to do just that—and Hans told him he could have a book put together in no time, to show for this impromptu support group he'd organized. Jeff glances at his hands, suddenly shy, then looks up at the rest of us with eyes full of emotion. "Maybe I could have helped him—if I could have freed up the time. Some hope."

Ellie tells the story of Charlene, an eight-year-old with sickle cell disease. It is wonderful to hear her tale told from a student's viewpoint, because I know Charlene well.

"When I first had her assigned to me," Ellie starts, "she'd come in with this cramping belly ache, and severe pains in her legs. She had been in for three lengthy admissions in the past year. This one was just before Christmas, so school was getting out. Just as all her friends were preparing for the celebrations, Charlene was stuck in a hospital bed on the end of an I.V. needle, getting the unwelcome gifts of morphine infusions and an antibiotic cocktail.

"When I checked her in, I had to be careful about sitting on her bed, because the weight of the blankets on her legs was painful." Ellie hesitates, and she too looks about to tear up. "But you know, that little kid, she never once complained about anything. Even when I had to stick her two or three times because her veins are so shot. She would just say, 'It's okay, doctor, I'll stay still.' And she did. Every day when I went to check on her, it was, 'I'm getting better.' And she would offer examples, like, 'It's easier making it to the bathroom,' and 'I ate all my grits today.' She would always want me to try cutting down on her pain meds, so she could be more awake, and we'd know if she was on the mend.

"But what really got me was, she was so *grateful* all the time. She'd say 'thank you, doctor,' even when all I could do was sit with her, try to cheer her up, and tell her she might get home for Christmas. She had a real 'attitude of gratitude.' Well, I soon found out she came by this honestly. Never a day when at least one family member wasn't there with her. Often it would be her grandma, so Mom could check on her other four kids before heading off to work, or even her teacher, who would have a couple of Charlene's siblings ride along so they could hang out with Charlene."

Amit, another student, hands Ellie a box of tissues. "Sorry, guys," Ellie tries to muster a grin through her tears, "I just felt real helpless, you know. And that little girl, she did as much for me as I could ever do for her."

"Not too much to apologize for, Ellie," I murmur. "It's a lovely story. Sometimes the only thing we can do—it's the best thing of all, mind—is spend time with our patients. Hang out with them, while they do their own healing. I found that out a long, long time ago. And you know what Voltaire said, 'The patient does the healing while the doctor takes the fee!'"

Ellie blows her nose and continues, "I went in to see her Christmas Day, even though I had the weekend off. There was only a handful of patients in the whole ward, mostly the real sick ones. But Charlene's whole family was there in her room, and Mom and the two youngest brothers had stayed over Christmas Eve night. Charlene had given the nurses gifts Mom had brought in, even one for me. A pretty merry Christmas, that was."

As we sit around on my floor, feeling our closeness—physical and emotional—it occurs to me that these beautiful and smart-as-whips doctors-to-be are perhaps hearing their own true voices for the first time. It is hard to put the meaning of holistic medicine into words: far better to show than to tell.

Before I take off for the holistic medical association gathering, I make a new friend in an unexpected quarter. Our College of Medicine's Dean, Allen Neims, invites me to join him at his early morning chat sessions. This proves nothing like the usual academic meetings I am in the habit of shunning. The ten or twelve of us seated along each side are clearly here to talk about *ourselves*. After introductions, each takes a turn to share something of our working or personal lives. More than once, Allen reminds us that what is said in this room stays right here. A neuroscientist, Lou Ritz, describes The Temple of the Universe, a yoga and meditation centre on six-hundred acres outside Gainesville, where he and his wife spend increasing amounts of time exploring their spiritual lives.

"Mickey Singer founded it back in 1975," he tells us. "He had this spiritual awakening, and decided to live alone in the woods and embrace a solitary spiritual life. He has bought up this rural land for preservation, and it turns out he's been a huge inspiration to lots of people. I've been wondering if we could start a program here in the medical school to explore the links between spirituality and health. I think Mickey would support it, and we could bring in speakers, maybe develop an elective course for students."

Allen responds enthusiastically. "That sounds like a lot of fun. Maybe there's a bit of money lying around here in the Dean's office that hasn't been earmarked!"

Allen and Lou and I get back together the following week to plan what we quickly dub the Center for Spirituality & Health. We come up with a simple mission statement—"to promote interdisciplinary teaching and research about spirituality and health"—and create our own website (www.spiritualityandhealth.ufl.edu). I leave feeling uplifted by having found like-minded souls—something sorely lacking in my professional life. And if I thought there weren't any like-minded physicians out there, my first day at the holistic medicine conference quickly puts me right. I am greeted at registration by exuberant men and women selling multicolored T-shirts with the organizational logo on them, the words "Hugs Heal" in bold capitals on the back. Putting words into action, the middle-aged balding guy who sold me my tee follows up with a welcoming hug.

"Rob Ivker. Great to see you here. I'm from Colorado. This your first time?"

"Yup. John Graham-Pole, from Florida. Looks like you guys are having fun!"

"That's the plan. I think I saw your name on the program?"

"Right. But there are a whole lot of other sessions I'll want to check out."

Over the next three days, I encounter several hundred physicians who have recognized the need to embrace a more holistic approach to caring for their patients. It goes well beyond vitamins and homeopathics. These men and women lead by example, exploring all kinds of ways for themselves and their staff to live healthier lifestyles. Each morning begins with either yoga or tai chi, then a healthy breakfast, checking in about our hopes for changing our working environments back home. On the last morning, Rob invites a group of about twenty of us older men to trek into the foothills of the White Mountains.

"We like to call ourselves 'sages,'" Rob tells us, "because the older women at the meeting are having their simultaneous gathering of 'crones.'"

After an invigorating walk we stop to rest on an outcrop of boulders, and Rob challenges each one of us. "Now, which day of the week do you take off from every kind of work activity? I'm not talking religion here, but which day do you take for your sabbatical?"

There is rueful laughter all round as we eye each other. The idea of taking a whole day every week to rest from our labors, to enjoy total "R and R," does seem laughable.

"All right, then," Rob continues, "which of you are willing to commit to taking a sabbatical from now on? Starting as soon as you get home? Because if we're serious about setting good examples for our patients, we need to really think about this. The evidence is well established—the medical profession is among the *least healthy* in our whole culture."

One or two of us start talking about how they might rearrange their working lives to move in the direction Rob is urging. But I can hardly look him in the eye, accustomed as I am to spending leisure hours poring over research papers, writing my own articles, putting the finishing touches to a grant application, or planning a new teaching course. And Sheila is even more dedicated to advancing her career. She often sleeps through Saturdays or Sundays after pulling a couple of all-nighters on a project with an urgent deadline. Rob's challenge has certainly given me food for thought as I head home to Florida.

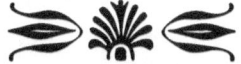

Chapter 9: *HOMECOMING*

A week after my return, I get a call out of the blue that makes me feel the stars are aligning as the universe ordered them. It's from Tim Bowen, the director of Hospice of North Central Florida.

"We've decided to add a hospice dedicated to children, and we'd like you to become its medical director. What do you think? We've got twenty adult beds, covering eighteen counties in northern Florida. It's a pretty big catchment area, as you can imagine. And your work would be largely home visiting, we wouldn't expect you to admit many children here."

I have no idea how Tim Bowen got my name, but the timing could hardly be better, because I had recently initiated a conversation with my department chairman, Terry Flotte, about establishing a palliative care service at Shands, and he'd made very supportive noises.

"Thanks for thinking of me. I'd be most interested—perhaps we can get together to talk?"

Tim and Bob McCollough, the hospice's medical director, and I meet for lunch to thrash out details. Although I've never met either before, they obviously knew a good bit about me and apparently satisfied themselves I'd be the right person. A week later I meet with Terry and my hematology-oncology chief, Steve Hunger, to discuss my future in the department. As I rehearse what I want to propose, I sense a chance to build on this synchronicity of events. My growing interest in the art of care and how the arts can create a more holistic environment, mesh with everything I have come to know about the growing field of palliative care. As soon as the three of us are settled in Terry's office, I announce my interest in working full-time in palliative care. I've come fully prepared with everything I can glean about such pediatric services around the country, which don't exist in Florida.

"It's not just children with cancer that can benefit. Our neonatologists, pulmonologists, I.C.U. guys, they all know of my interests and are talking to me about consulting on their patients. Now our Florida hospice has asked me to set up their children's hospice program, so this seems the perfect opportunity to build a joint service between our two organizations."

A lengthy pause, then Steve comments, "Well, I don't think I've too much more to contribute if this is to be your full-time commitment, John. But we'll be happy to make referrals to you." With that, he makes his excuses and leaves us to work out the details of my new position. Terry tells me he can lay his hands on the money for a nurse practitioner, a half-time social worker, and continued funding for Rebecca Brown, whom I'd hired earlier as a music therapist and pastoral counselor. Meanwhile, Tim and Bob have assigned two nurses, another part-time social worker, and a grief counselor to work with me, and Bob lets me know he will sit in on rounds until I'm familiar with how things run.

As I leave Terry's office, I reflect that my career has taken a quantum leap. I'll never again attend those national oncology group shindigs, and I feel only relief. Whatever I have contributed to my long-ago chosen field of serving children with cancer and their families has given me many years of fulfillment, but there are many young guns eager to fill my shoes. I've had this "been there, done that" feeling for some time, so it seems high time to move over and start exploring new pastures. As I glance at my publications over the last five years I realize they all concern the *art* of my profession rather than its *science*.

After my initial elation at my new professional autonomy, I come down to earth with the need to justify my continuing full professor's salary. Tim sets up meetings with the hospice's finance department, bringing me face-to-face with my naiveté around the big wide world of billing for services. Having worked in four university hospitals over nearly forty years, I am only vaguely aware of what goes on in offices whose job revolves around generating money. I've been especially protected by working with children with life-threatening illnesses, because no hospital administrator will ever turn away such children for lack of ability to pay. But hospice has to rely on strictly limited financial support from charitable and government sources, so it comes down to charging for our services. The whole thing is a steep learning curve, especially because it is hard to get my head around billing the families of children for whom modern medicine has no curative therapies to offer. Bob McCollough is sympathetic but gently points out that everyone is largely salaried by the income generated by billing. So charge I must.

It isn't quite such a steep learning curve at Shands. Terry clearly sees my new palliative care division as an investment that is unlikely to generate much financial return in the short term. But only from painstaking research through physician billing codes do I figure out how to bring in an income. I find to my astonishment that I can charge not only for length of time at the bedside, but for services provided away from the bedside, too. These range from educating hospital staff to developing palliative protocols, from admin meetings to making house calls. The fly in the ointment is it all demands written documentation on appropriate forms, plus exact measurement of the time requirement. A lot of paperwork—with a sudden dearth of secretarial support. But I am encouraged to find a focus on palliation rather than cure leads to significant savings in pharmacy, laboratory, and I.C.U. costs, and I stress this during my consultations, which start to pick up quickly.

I feel I should somehow be an expert on dealing with the death of a child. After all, since five-year-old Audrey's death back in Norwich in 1969 about half the many hundreds of children I've cared for have died. Chests from adult-sized to tiny I'll never again sound, tummies I'll never again prod and palpate. I remember as a resident doctor I had sat for a few wordless minutes with Audrey's mother after pronouncing her daughter dead. How much training do students and residents get in being with the dying or bereaved? Close to fifty years ago, suffering my own terrible bereavement with Mummy's death, I remember only the numbness that afflicted me for over twenty years. I had to wait until I was in my mid-thirties before meeting Barbara, who somehow knew how to release the floodgates and started my own healing journey. A transition so profound it affected my whole life course. What have I learned from all that that I can pass on to others?

As I prepare myself to be the constant fellow traveler with death and those about to enter its portals, I'm drawn to C.S. Lewis's book, *A Grief Observed*, and how he describes his bereavement after his wife died: "No one ever told me that grief felt so like fear . . . same fluttering in the stomach . . . restlessness . . . like mildly drunk, or concussed." Writing about his own grief over Helen's death seems to console him. "One never meets just Cancer . . . one only meets each hour or moment that comes. All manner of ups and downs . . . bad spots in our best times, many good ones in our worst." I think about how hugely helpful it's been to write requiems for my patients, albeit they are a pale shadow of the losses their families suffer.

Maybe the real essence of the work of serving the very ill and dying, especially parents, is to help them uncover the meaning behind Lewis's words, take comfort from those best times, as long as they and their child can be together on earth. My full-time job for the past thirty years has been oncology and hematology, perceived by my peers as a medical scientist. Caring for dying patients has never been part of our training curriculum. The interest I've nurtured in palliative care and all that goes with it has bloomed essentially in secret. Somewhere along the line, care for the dying has consumed my awareness, without mentors, as with many twists and turns in my professional life. How did I happen on writing poetry to cope with daily work challenges? What brought me to explore the psychology of childhood illnesses, and thus my meeting Sheila? More serendipity. Now I've found fellow travelers: physicians championing holistic approaches to care for all, including ourselves. And most pivotal of all: uniting with all my artist-teacher companions as we uncovered art's boundless healing power.

So many digressions and byways from the conventional path of a children's cancer specialist, that carrying card that secured all my faculty appointments and ultimately led to my tenure as full professor. Maya Angelou said, "Uh oh . . . I've run a game on everybody, and they're going to find me out." So how many have I had to fool to arrive at my present situation?

One thing has guided and nourished me since I joined the company of Quakers twenty-five years ago: a commitment to bring body, mind, and soul to work each day. Quakers say "there is that of God in everyone," that it's vital to find the still small space in each person, in each encounter. Not easy when modern medicine's heady considerations consume me and the patients themselves can quickly vanish from view. But if I can bring a fraction of that meditative silence of Friends worship to each bedside, then these moments can feel more like communion than conversation. Children with illness that may take them before they have fastened roots in our earth may be closer to spirit than grown-ups, able to draw more easily on its resource. I just got an email from Gena, a deeply spiritual woman of thirty-three married to a doctor of theology, Justin. Acute leukemia almost took Gena's life at eighteen months. But her spirit had shone from her as parents, Dee and Gene, lit candles and prayed through their daughter's first night in my care. Gena writes in her email: "Nothing is wasted, not even our pain. God uses it for a greater good."

Soon after my new position as medical director of palliative care is announced, a colleague whom Steve had just hired fresh from fellowship stops me in the atrium.

"You remember that sixteen-year-old girl, Ella, with non-Hodgkin's lymphoma you diagnosed two months back? I'm managing her care now, and she's in bad shape. Could you get involved again?"

I remember Ella instantly. She had almost died the day we admitted her in deep shock with her mother beseeching me to "for God's sake, do something, doctor," even as we struggled to draw her daughter back from the brink. On top of her widespread cancer, she had developed *pseudomonas* septicemia from an infected belly stud. It wasn't until the following afternoon I judged Ella ready to hear the awful news, sitting at her bedside across from still panicky Mom.

"There's no easy way to tell you this, Ella, but you need to know everything that's going on. What's happened is, you've got cancer—a cancer we call lymphoma. We've already started giving you treatment to get you back completely healthy again."

"What treatment?"

"We call it chemotherapy—chemo for short. Drugs to kill your cancer."

"Am I going to die?"

Her apparent calm and her direct questioning told me there was no hiding anything from this young woman.

"I don't think so, Ella. But our treatment will make you feel rotten, as bad for a while as your cancer."

"How come you didn't ask *me* about this treatment?"

"Ella, you were really out of it last night, and we needed to start right away. You're also a minor, so it's your parents who have to give us permission."

She had been silent then, but I sensed she didn't put too much faith in what her new doctor was up to. The treatment proved perhaps worse than her disease, pulling Ella back to fragile life while its horrid toxicity crushed her adolescent beauty. Within weeks, a further hideous insult hit, which is why my colleague has asked me to get involved again—but in my new palliative care persona. The cancer penetrates Ella's spinal cord, paralyzing her from the waist down, so she can no longer move or feel her legs or empty her bladder and bowel on her own.

Scanning her medical notes to update myself, my eye catches on the resident doctor's dispassionate chart note for what would prove Ella's final admission. *Caucasian female, 16 years; known non-Hodgkin's, admitted with recurrence. Prior admits for chemo admin., fever, neutropenia, rule-out sepsis. Physical exam positive for scalp alopecia, healing mouth ulcers, extensive acne face and neck, paralysis and sensory loss from waist down, bladder catheter in place, multiple venipuncture scars, grade II abdominal striae, minimal muscle bulk.* All in all, a physical wreck—and no doubt an emotional one, too—but nothing in this terse clinical note pays even lip service to this. I am filled with anger at the bloodless way our young doctors are taught to report on their patients, giving way to profound sorrow at this whole senseless tragedy. Why do such ghastly things happen to such beautiful young people?

Meanwhile, her parents are increasingly desperate, my oncologist colleague tells me. "They're a bit—make that a lot—out of touch with reality. Talking about taking Ella to Sloan Kettering for some highly experimental therapy, even exploring heavily touted treatments in Mexico. When I asked them if they'd talked to their daughter, Mom responded that Ella was barely sixteen years old, so in no position to make her own decisions. At that point, I felt this was getting out of my league, and that if anyone could help the situation it was you."

I feel an unexpected warmth at this compliment from Steve Hunger's newest recruit. Maybe there is something to be said for my having gone around the block a few times in the past few decades. As I make my way to Ella's isolation room I know better than to prepare any speeches. Winging it is an under-appreciated resource, especially if I remember to listen a whole lot more than talk. I meet her mother right inside the door, along with a man who introduces himself as Ella's dad.

"We need to talk, doctor," her mother starts right in. "I know you've been asked to come just to make Ella comfy, that you've all given up on her getting better. But we—my husband and I—want to take her to Sloan Kettering. We're just not ready to give up."

She is growing increasingly agitated, and I quickly abandon any idea of sitting down for a quiet chat in the family room. "Mrs Dickson, my colleague filled me in on everything. And I know you want to do all you possibly can for Ella. But can we talk after I've had a chance to chat with your daughter?"

"Doctor, she won't listen to us—she doesn't have any fight left." Her mother is crying freely, while Ella's dad makes awkward efforts to comfort her. "Can't we get a court order or something if she goes on refusing? We've just got to do *something*!"

I am unprepared for just how sick Ella has become. Her resident has told me she has pneumonia—no surprise given her diaphragmatic muscles can't be firing properly because of her paralysis, but I hadn't expected to see her struggling for every breath. She is perilously close to needing a ventilator to take over her breathing and help her get enough oxygen, as well as much needed rest. I kneel close by her bedside to talk while her parents sit stiffly and apart behind me.

"Ella, Dr. Sampson asked me to come see you. To see what we can do to make you comfy. It's real hard for you to breathe, isn't it? Your mom and dad want you to get different chemo, but we would have to put you on a breathing machine..."

"I'm not going to get better, am I?" She pauses every few words to catch her breath but holds my look. I lean in even closer, wanting to keep the talk just between the two of us.

"No, Ella, no, I don't think you are. But I can help you relax, breathe easier, not hurt any more."

She moves a pale hand a few inches towards mine. I take the cue and grasp it, feel its fragility.

"Don't want more chemo." Her breath is ever more labored, words weakening. "No other hospital. No breathing machine." She stops, then, "But... can you stay with me?"

"Yes, I can stay with you," I answer without thought. "Can I just talk to Mom and Dad a bit first?"

I turn to where her parents had been sitting, only to find they have moved to the window bay. Dad has his arms wrapped around his wife while she sobs quietly against his shoulder. I move over and squat awkwardly between them.

"It's all right—do whatever you think is best, doctor. We don't want her hurting anymore."

A huge weight lifts from me. Knowing the futility of travelling to New York or Mexico, or anywhere else, for some highly experimental therapy, I breathe a silent prayer of thanks as I move back to Ella's side.

"Ella, I'm going to stay right here with you."

Her nurse comes in quietly and stands at the door. I explain everything and ask her to get her resident doctor *asap*, so he can write up the necessary medicines, then I settle in. I end up camping by the top of her bed for thirty-six hours, dozing and waking, my right hand always clasping her left. The morphine and Ativan infusion succeeds in slowing her breathing and easing her anxiety, and she sleeps for longer and longer spells. Her oxygen levels hover perilously low despite her airtight mask, but mercifully we don't have to raise the issue of the ventilator again. Sometimes I doze off myself. The nurses bring me in food trays, just as if I am part of the family, though I have little appetite. Her parents spend most of their time in our social worker's room. They are no longer fighting the decision—had perhaps realized it was their daughter's to make. But the pain of watching her die by inches is too hard for them to endure for long.

Ella has a small blackboard propped against her knees and rouses every so often to scrawl a few words. *Not scared . . . no machines . . . thanks . . .* She is adamant she wants to stay as awake and aware as possible, her spirit somehow sustaining her even as she suffers physical anguish. As she fades, her face takes on a look of ease, even of grace. The silences are broken only by the sound of her deepening, slowing breaths. I could be at a Quaker meeting for worship. Close to the end, I sense something almost physical passing between us. As though she is shedding her dying cells into my breath, while I am breathing my own healthy ones back into her. As if I'm carrying something deathless within her out into our temporal world, while she transports shreds of my earthly self to rest with her in eternity.

I make my first trip out to the hospice in northwest Gainesville, and as I introduce myself at the front desk, the receptionist points to the big glass window behind her.

"Meet our new arrivals, doctor! Though they've got a very different reason for being here than most of our occupants!"

I look out at the shaded patch of grass and fallen pine needles and am astonished to see two full-sized turkey vultures eying me from beyond the glass. Their interest quickly returns to their primary preoccupation—two cream-colored eggs lying close together between them. There is no sign of any nest, and the only protection for this unlikely family is some scrubby palmetto bushes.

"They've only been there a week and apparently it'll take six weeks for the chicks to hatch. Dad seems to spend as much time with them as Mom. Very attentive they are!"

"Well, this is a new experience for me. It'll make my trips out here especially fun."

As I join my new staff, I reflect on the happy irony of these creatures choosing a hospice to bring new life into the world. Paula and Cendra are my two nurses, and a social worker and chaplain are assigned to work with us. The first question that surfaces is what to call ourselves. After lots of creative suggestions, Paula dreams up the name, *Pegasus*, and we have fun designing a logo to capture the image of the mythical winged horse. Then Cendra asks how I see my new job and I jump right in.

"I've dug up some bleak facts to support Tim Bowen's and Terry Flotte's decision. It turns out there are 400,000 children—babies to teens—living in our country with incurable illnesses, and 55,000 die each year. About 3,000 children in Florida alone, over a 100 at Shands. But many aren't included in the 400,000 because many are sudden infant deaths, accidents, or suicides. The real kicker is that less than one percent of these children ever receive hospice care."

"So what are we going to do about all this?" Cendra looks impatient with all these facts and figures. "Shouldn't we be coming up with our own plans?"

"Yup, you're right. I'm thinking like an administrator already—doing a needs assessment. Okay, so what do we want Pegasus to look like?"

We spend the next hour brainstorming while Paula writes on a flip chart that has appeared from somewhere. The first draft looks like this:

Our focus—every child's comfort and quality of life

Suffering can be physical, psychological, social, or spiritual—or all four at once

Everyone's needs are unique, not least because of difference in ages—from newborns to college students

We want to offer these children the very best care setting—hopefully at home, but hospice or hospital when needed

These illnesses affect not just children, but whole families, even whole communities

Cure and care are far from mutually exclusive—it's not either/or but both/and

We must offer round-the-clock care, especially to children who stay at home

And never forget respite and bereavement care for families, including perhaps

a camp for siblings
Vital to build in rituals, like memorial services and annual remembrances
And we must look after ourselves, and each other, as allies and friends

"It's quite a bit," Paula comments, which gets us laughing at this marvelous understatement. "Okay, time for a tea break—we've been at this for two hours. If all our staff meetings go this long, we'll never get any real work done!"

The thought of house calls jumps into my mind—something not yet mentioned. This could add hugely to my time commitment, given we are meant to cover eighteen north Florida counties. But I feel a thrill of excitement as my mind jumps back to my house calls with Uncle Ken—my very first exposure to my future profession. Nobody is telling me how to spend my working time—and doesn't seeing my patients and their families in their own homes symbolize that "quiet art" Virgil spoke of? Only I won't be sitting with the wives and children while the man of the house breathes his last. Our children will be, yes, incurably ill, but by no means at the point of death. We'll have time to enjoy each other's company, make memories, come to know the child's and family's ultimate wishes.

Cendra takes me to meet sixteen-year-old Alicia at her home twenty-five miles northeast of Gainesville. She has a slow-growing brain tumor, has gone through extensive surgery and radiation, and chemotherapy isn't an option. Her life is in no immediate danger, but she's quite disabled and spends her time in her wheelchair in front of the T.V. Dad works full-time as an electrician and Mom stays home to care for Alicia while raising two other school-aged children and taking in part-time work as a seamstress. Alicia's biggest problem is she craves food constantly, probably because of the tumor's location around a small section of her mid-brain—the hypothalamus—which governs a person's appetite. It never seems to switch off, which isn't helped by her corticosteroids, which are appetite stimulants. Her mom has to give them whenever Alicia shows signs of pressure building up in her brain—early-morning headache and throwing up—because of the tumor swelling unpredictably.

Mom introduces me to her daughter as she prepares tea. It's hard to wrest Alicia's attention away from the T.V., but she greets me with a huge beam and grasps my hand hard with her one good hand. Cendra and I sit ourselves on each side sipping our teacups, and the nurse quickly shows her skills at holding her attention.

"You've been on a cruise, haven't you, Alicia?"

Cendra has already filled me in that the Childrens' Wish Foundation had sponsored this all-expenses-paid trip for Alicia and her family.

"Yes, yes, yes. It was *fun*. A big boat."

"Did your little sister come, too? And your brother?"

"Yes. And Daddy." More beaming.

"What was the best part, Alicia?" Cendra is grinning impishly, like they are sharing some private joke. Alicia simply beams back.

"How was the food?" I prompt, pretty sure I'm onto what the fun is about.

Now Alicia is giggling like she knows she's been caught doing something naughty. Cendra wraps her arm around her and they dissolve in mirth. Mom is laughing, too, though trying to hold back.

"There were six restaurants, doctor," she tells me. "After the first day I gave up trying to keep Alicia away. It was like an all-day guided tour—she knew each one within a day, and what they had to offer. I can't hardly find clothes for her to wear any more. She must have got the whole idea of the cruise from the T.V.—that they were food city!"

"So a good time was had by all, eh?"

"I guess so, doctor—we gained a few pounds ourselves. We did get Alicia walking around the deck some with the other children, And they had the best time—lots of stuff organized for them. It was hard getting them off the boat!"

I check through my list of relevant issues—Alicia's symptoms and signs, her meds and her compliance with them, how Mom and Dad and Alicia's sibs are coping, financial worries, and so forth. Mom is at apparent peace with her situation. I mention the idea of respite—that we could admit Alicia to hospice for a few days to give everyone a break, but Mom looks almost shocked we'd consider such a thing. As I write out the necessary refill prescriptions, Mom takes us back to an unforgettable happening on the cruise.

"We had this big scare, doctor. We set an alarm at night that connects through to our room from Alicia's, lets us know if she gets out of bed. We thought we had it all hooked up between the kids' and our cabin, but it didn't work this one time. I woke up in the middle of the night knowing something was amiss. Mom's instinct, I guess. Sure enough, Alicia is gone from her bed, while the other kids are sleeping like a hurricane wouldn't wake 'em. I rouse my husband and we start searching around, finally come on this cleaner who says maybe she fell overboard someplace, which gets even me rattled. We're checking every deck, most of them with scarcely a light on. But the top is all lit up and the restaurant is open for business. So who should be setting right there by the buffet table alongside the waiter but our Alicia. Stuffing herself, she was, with the waiter chatting away to her! I guess he thinks she's got the okay to be up here—her being almost a grown-up. Heavenly Jesus, I couldn't stop crying, seeing my little girl not just safe but having the time of her life!"

On the drive back to Gainesville, Cendra and I reflect on what we've witnessed. "How long do you think she can live, Doctor John?"

"Well, she's sure happy, and Mom is utterly devoted, so she's getting the very best care. I don't see any point in repeating her C.A.T. scans—but from what I can see, she could go on trucking for months. Who knows, years, I guess?"

My new medical practice is a one-eighty switch from struggling to pull patients back from the brink of death with our latest chemo cocktails. "Pegasus therapy" is everything we brainstormed: care and comfort for our children and families as long as they need us. Which can mean doing little beyond listening over a cup of tea, linking our hearts to theirs. Bob McCollough and I attend the national hospice meeting in Houston, and the first morning Elizabeth Kubler-Ross is introduced, famous for her work on the way many people seem to prepare for death—the five stages of grief. Now elderly and frail, she is escorted to the podium in a wheel chair. She speaks for a few minutes before receiving a standing ovation from her several hundred listeners, which lasts at least as long as her speech.

Most sessions are devoted to clinical trials of the latest medication for pain or other symptoms, understandably focused on care of older adults, so I am delighted to find a gathering of those working with children. Of the twenty-odd who show up, only Boston Children's Hospital seems to have a well-established program. Back home, I suggest to Melissa, my nurse practitioner, that we go to Boston to learn from their expertise. A phone call to Joanne Wolfe, the clinical director, confirms that she is quite used to short visits from colleagues setting up their own children's palliative care units. We spend our time making daily rounds with the staff, sitting in on teaching seminars, discussing new consults, and talking with parents of Joanne's patients. Melissa spends much of her time with the nurse-coordinator, and the two of us start thinking about how to implement everything we have learned. One thing our visit confirms is the need for champions among our fellow physicians and nurses if children are to get referred in time for us to be of real service. A consult for "terminal pain management" received a few hours before death offers no such opportunity.

The day after we get home, I'm back on the road to meet eleven-year-old Warren and his family, who live in a mobile home close to the airport. I had known Warren since I had first treated his bone cancer, with apparent success, but about a year afterwards it had reappeared in both lungs. He had gone on to get so-called second-line drug treatments, but with little effect, so his mother made the brave decision to have him home for his remaining time. I was happy I would again be looking after him, even in these sad circumstances. Cendra tells me his dad is working in Georgia, laying an extension to Interstate I-95, and can only get home at weekends, but Warren's three teenage sisters are there after school to help Mom, while spending time with their much-loved brother. Mom has taught them to cook, and they prepare the evening meal I get to sample during our visit. Warren is on around-the-clock morphine, supplemented by special care from Grandma, long known as a powerful natural healer. Chief among these healing remedies is a prayer ritual conducted three times daily with the whole family—Cendra and me included this time.

My only medical task is to go over Warren's care with Mom and Cendra and renew his prescriptions. I figure out his average daily costs in full-time hospice at $125, while during his earlier hospitalizations at Shands his bills had often run over $1,000 a day. Since there are few medical issues and Warren is sleeping peacefully on the mattress made up for him on the floor of the front room, I spend my time between the afternoon prayer ritual and supper getting acquainted with the family. I quiz the girls about their homework, only to find that most of it goes straight over my head. Mom makes a point of acquainting me with three generations of the family, framed photos of whom grace every conceivable surface. On my next visit, Mom has moved up a planned family reunion to make sure everyone gets to say their goodbyes, and I meet about thirty teens or twenty-somethings hanging out in the driveway drinking beer or coke. Warren has roused himself for the occasion and recognizes most of his cousins and uncles and aunts, even if he has trouble with their names.

My final visit comes three days later when I get a call from Warren's mom, who tells me calmly that her son has just passed, and that Cendra and our social worker are on their way. When I get there, Warren is propped on pillows on his parents' bed with the whole family gathered at his bedside. After I've signed the death certificate, Mom hugs me as she sobs quietly.

"Doc, I want a photo, just of you and Warren. You were so good to him. Could you maybe climb up on his bed?"

I treasure that picture of Warren and me, though I don't show it around to many of my colleagues.

But if Warren's passing could be described as "a good death," some can only be described as awful. I am asked to consult on Jake, a fourteen-year-old on a ventilator in the I.C.U., whose longstanding lung problems are finally getting the better of him. The staff have debated long and hard about whether to use the ventilator. Jake's recent deterioration was the end result of a steadily downhill course. But his grandma/guardian had the final word and insisted on what many felt was a futile course of action. They had called me in to help Grandma come to terms with the situation, but it quickly became apparent that there wasn't any reasoning with this hard-scrabble family. Late in the evening after my second visit I get called back up to the unit.

"John, can you see if you can help?" The nurse sounds pretty desperate on the phone, with a lot of hoopla in the background. "Jake's E.T. tube is out, he's coughing blood and putting up a huge fight."

I come upon a scene of bedlam. The attending physician, several nurses, and the respiratory therapist are surrounding Jake's bed, the floor awash with leaking bags of saline, penciled records of bellowed orders, dropped syringes, and torn-off E.K.G. strips. As I ease myself to the bedside, Jake is resisting everyone's efforts to reintubate him, spluttering between bloody coughs, "Let me effing die! Let me effing die!" Then, "I'm not your effing sweetheart!" at one of the nurses doing her level best to calm him. Grandma is meanwhile screaming abuse at all and sundry, spots me, and sees me as a good target.

"If he dies, you're going too!"

After fifteen minutes more of this madhouse scene, Jake's efforts finally cease enough for the resident to reintubate him, only for the E.K.G. monitor to flatline. The staff goes through the ritual of cardiopulmonary resuscitation, more to show that everything possible has been done, before calling off the whole tragic fiasco. Grandma is finally escorted out of the unit, and I make one more attempt to comfort her. Her response is to underline her earlier threat: "We'll get you, don't you worry, boy. We'll get you!" By this time, there are several security guards on the scene, and Maggie, the senior one and a longtime friend, takes me aside.

"John, we've gotta take threats like this seriously. I'm gonna see you safely off the premises. Go straight home and stay there till I call you."

My two-weeks unlooked-for vacation finally ends, but it's a long time before I feel entirely comfortable walking the corridors at night.

The following week, I make a trip with visiting friends to show them the old fishing village of Cedar Key, sixty miles southwest of Gainesville. We are halfway there when my pager rings.

"Sorry to bother you, Dr. John, but I'm out at Marie's house. You know, the little girl with the brain tumor. She's getting horrid headaches, and I need a stat order to up her I.V. morphine dose. The pressure must be building up in her head."

This is a first: ordering I.V. narcotics over the phone to my new nurse from fifty-odd miles away.

"What's she on?"

"Two mg every four hours—I want to go straight to three."

"I agree, and give her another milligram in ten minutes if it's not cutting it."

We are on our way back from Cedar Key when Cendra calls again.

"I've been trying to reach you—you must have been in a dead zone. Anyway, she's sleepy but writhing about. I want to go up some more."

"Sorry, Cendra, I was all the way to Cedar Key. I'll join you as soon as I've dropped my friends back. So what weight is she?"

"Just over thirty pounds—say fifteen kilograms."

I do quick calculations. The usual single dose of I.V. morphine is 0.1mg/kg, so we're already at over twice the normal dose. But what do we have to lose? Marie has been fading quickly, and on my last visit her parents were more than ready to let her go.

"Let's go with four mg and another two every thirty minutes."

Forty minutes later, Cendra reports Marie is still moaning and thrashing, even though she is barely rousable from her coma. "And the local pharmacy has only one I.V. morphine dose left, Dr. John. There's a van coming from

Shands with further supplies. I don't know how long she can last." I detect a hint of desperation in this calm and competent nurse's voice.

"I should be with you in twenty minutes. Give her five mg every ten till I'm there."

When I finally make it, I know at a glance Marie is at last at peace. Mom is cradling her little girl in her arms while Dad and Cendra hold Mom between them.

"She's been gone only five minutes, John. It was peaceful at the end."

It's the first time Cendra has dropped the "Dr." I reflect that between us we had brought this little girl's life to a quite intentional end. How the lawyers would see this scenario I'm not sure, but there aren't any around, and Mom's last words leave me in no doubt we had done the absolutely right thing in these tragic circumstances.

"Thank you, doctor, and Cendra, for helping us, for giving our dear little girl relief from her suffering."

It was my nurse—in the tradition of so many Florence Nightingales—who had done all the heavy lifting in giving loving and skillful care to this family and their little girl.

A week later, there is a message waiting for me after making rounds from someone called Leo Rooney, a vaguely familiar name. I check my patient records, and confirm we had sent sixteen-year-old Leo Junior home to hospice care two years earlier. I remember our conversation the last time the family had brought him to my clinic. He was prematurely wise in the ways of the world—children with cancer seem to grow up fast—and he always sat in on family conferences. It was clear who was calling the shots nowadays about what was best for him.

"Leo, I don't think we should plan more visits. We've been over everything, and there's really no other treatments can help. You're a very long way from us down there in West Palm and you've got a great family doc can look after everything. I'll be checking in on the phone regularly."

"Okay, doc," Leo responded. "You've given it your best shot, so now I'll just have to try some other things."

And God knows, there are plenty of options out there. I rarely meet a patient who hasn't checked out the Internet, or heard from a friend about a new cure they've heard about. But Leo would for sure need a miracle to last more than a few weeks. Two years on, as I review Leo's chart, I notice it would have been his eighteenth birthday today, though he was surely long dead. Perhaps Leo Senior had felt the need to call on what must be a painful anniversary for the family. I dial the number, ask for Mr. Rooney.

"Which one?"

I'm caught short. Just how many Leo Rooneys are there at this number? Then I realize this is a young man's voice. He saves me from more confusion.

"Hi, doc—yup, it's me! Surprised to hear from me? I just got a new car for my birthday, and I'll be heading up your way. Starting at U.F. in the Fall, the Cancer Society gave me a full scholarship."

"Hey, this is just great, Leo," I stammer after I'm over my initial surprise. "So how are you doing? You sound great!"

"Sure am, doc. I was thinking maybe you could arrange a C.A.T. scan to check if there's anything left to see. Just curious, you know."

You're not the only one, I think to myself, but don't voice the thought. The scan shows some residual scarring in the areas of Leo's cancer in his leg and lungs, where it had spread two years earlier, but nothing more. In due course, he enrolls in our Engineering department and becomes a spokesperson for cancer in the young. Meanwhile, I do research on what has been written about miracle cures. It turns out an International Medical Commission of Lourdes was established in 1947, after evidence came to light that a few terminally ill people who had made the trip over the past hundred years to the Shrine of Our Lady of Lourdes in the Pyrenees had undergone such cures. The Commission was entrusted with identifying such cases on the grounds of hard-and-fast scientific scrutiny. There have been some six-thousand claims of cures, with over sixty meeting the Commission's very rigid criteria. So whatever modern medical biostatisticians might have to say about this, Albert Einstein put it best: "Not everything that counts can be counted." Would this august body of medical scientists classify Leo as a miracle cure? Well, they defer to the Church to make those pronouncements, but he's certainly satisfied me.

In November 2006, I break my plans to friends and colleagues to retire when I hit sixty-five in a few months. "Forty years since I started internship—seems like a good time."

"Well, you've got to give a last lecture," Mary Fukuyama, a sociologist friend says. "Hold up the tradition."

I have never heard of about-to-retire professors giving this last lecture, but I'm taken with the idea.

"We'll have a party afterwards," Lou adds, which clinches it.

I am astonished to find a packed house in the main lecture hall of the health sciences center. I recognize everyone facing me in the front two rows, but beyond this I pick out only a scattering of familiar faces. I'm even more astounded when the whole hall rises for a standing ovation as Allen Neims introduces me. I feel close to tears to find he has surfaced—who knows where from—pictures of my early childhood, including one of Weston-super-Mare sands, complete with donkeys. I struggle to compose myself in response to this tribute. "I haven't even said anything yet," is all I can come up with.

"Okay, so I'm going to talk a bit about how science and art complement each other in modern medicine. Freud said poetry drinks at streams not yet accessible to science. And Jonah Lehrer, in *Proust was a Neuroscientist*, shows how literature, music and visual art often precede science in uncovering the core workings of our brains. From his Prelude: 'By expressing our actual experience, the artist reminds us . . . no map of matter will ever explain the immateriality of our consciousness.' Epstein speaks about explicit quantifiable knowledge—what we call science—and tacit intuitive knowledge—let's call that art. Medical knowledge is provable with statistical certainty but much of our clinical practice relies on the purely personal experiences of givers and receivers of care. The mother of a teenager with advanced cancer asked me to explain his condition to him. Here's an extract from "The Color of Grief," a poem I wrote later to try to make sense of our conversation.

> *I press my body towards him, chair hiccupping on the*
> *new-laid Cancer Center carpeting; his bolts, reflexive,*
> *back into itself, eyes slipping in black-to-white deference,*
> *head drooping subjugate to my words, tongue licking at*
> *one boulder tear rolling furtive down a young man's cheeks.*

"This encounter brought up several questions for me: *What did my patient understand of his illness? How close a relationship can there be between two people separated so widely in age, race, and education? Was there anything else I could have said? In the end, how much value was I to this boy or his family?*

"Spying just one infinitely reluctant tear told me my patient understood something from my faltering words of his situation. But the space between us felt no closer at the end than at the start of our conversation. What was planned as an agreement on our next course of action became a stumbling one-sided speech. Medical science could supply answers to this boy's diagnosis, treatment and prognosis; but he couldn't, or wouldn't, pose the questions."

I continue my talk, offering examples of how in medicine, science and art can sometimes complement and sometimes conflict, then draw my conclusions.

"It's no accident we use the same word, *art*, to describe creating works of beauty and function and offering skilled, loving care to those in need. We caregivers try simultaneously to offer the very best of modern biomedicine while creating something artful from our intuitive in-the-moment skills. Cicely Saunders, founder of our modern hospice movement, said the best palliative care entails close human relationships, built through 'efficient loving care,' defined as a blend of knowledge, skill, and empathy.

"In trying to eliminate confounds and observer bias, medicine too often discounts the wealth of cultural and psychosocial experiences our patients bring with them. There may always be in medicine a divide between art and science—Eliot's 'silence between two waves of the sea'—but I hope in forty years of teaching, research, and clinical practice I've succeeded a little in closing that space."

People who are bereaved have been writing letters to their beloved dead since the time of Egypt's Old Kingdom, twenty-five-hundred years B.C. A month after my retirement, I write a letter to my mother, now dead fifty-three years.

> *Dear Mummy,*
> *High time I wrote you! The last letter I actually posted would have been from boarding school—more than fifty years ago. Yesterday, I was thinking about you and having a good cry—I guess grief lasts a lifetime. Maybe there haven't been many people I've really trusted since.*
> *But—65 years young and happier than ever! You'd be proud, and sure let me know it—like when I won that prize for Latin or that little silver cup at the school sports. Well, I just retired after forty years of doctoring, and about twenty years ago*

I finally figured out my course was subconsciously set the moment I first heard you'd died. Uncle Ken always tried to talk me out of being a doctor, and I could never come up with why I was so set on it. After all, I hated science in school! But I know now it was no accident I chose first oncology, then pediatrics. Your death made me declare a twelve-year-old's war on cancer. And after my miserable adolescence I lost my heart to the first sick child I saw—though it was scary as hell at first.

It still astounds me no one told me you were dead until three days afterwards. Looking back, I'm sure that lack of candor left an enduring mark on my whole career, and we're still avoiding the truth when we talk to our patients. So I want to tell you a bit of what I've learned about telling patients and families the truth, because I've been dwelling on this ever since they finally got around to letting me know what happened to you. The last four years, I've been a children's hospice doctor. People often ask me why—and lately I've been figuring that one out, too. I came back to Barts ten years after graduating as Britain's first full-time pediatric oncologist. Amazing to think the first chemo ever given for cancer was given to a little boy in Boston less than thirty years before—that child would be the same age as me if he'd lived.

It was the universally held view, in 1960's British medical circles at least, that telling the patient outright what was wrong with them—putting a name to their illness—would throw them into such a crisis it would quickly kill them. So silence was maintained by all. My very first week, this radiation oncologist asked me to see a patient I'll call Brian, whom he'd been treating for a widespread bone cancer. Did my new chemotherapy treatments have anything to offer, he wondered?

One look at Brian's X-rays told me his time was terribly short, and that any drugs I might offer would buy him a couple of months tops. When I went into his room, he was stretched out on a gurney in obvious pain, his parents on either side. It wasn't till I came closer, and our eyes met, that I realized abruptly that this whole scenario was an uncharted sea for me. I'd never had to tell a patient I had little beyond a little comfort to offer, let alone utter that spectral "D" word. I'm sure no one way back in the 1950's spoke directly of death with you; and it flashed on me that in all the conversations I'd witnessed between senior doctors and patients I had never seen real candor shown. None had even talked to us privately about how such dialogues should go; it just wasn't in the teaching curriculum.

But here I was, and here the buck stopped. I couldn't duck the truth and be true to myself. My first intuition was that I needed to talk to Brian directly, not just to his parents about him; so I pulled my chair up close, laid a hand on his forearm, and asked him how his treatments had been so far. Had they helped his pain? (It didn't look like it). He was hard to draw out till I asked when he was last home, and what he enjoyed doing. He loosened up a little, mentioned friends who came around, managed a wry grin about missing so much school. After a bit, I brought his parents in on the conversation, asking them what Dr. S. had told them. They were awkward talking freely in front of Brian, but when they saw I wasn't in a rush to leave and was encouraging them to open up a little, things started to flow. That dreaded word "cancer" came up for the first time between the three of them. Did anyone ever use that word with you, I wonder, Mummy?

For my part, I was having another, happier epiphany: listening was a whole lot easier than talking. I had time to sense not just the understanding but the emotional temperature between the three of them—and time to frame my own approach. I started reflecting back for them the sequence of Brian's illness, and what it really meant for a treatment to stop working. I told them all about chemotherapy, what they could reasonably expect, and at what expense in terms of side effects. I let each bit of this sink in, while giving myself time to breathe and take in their response. I told them they had choices, must weigh things between them, not rush their decision. And I told them I'd be happy to look after Brian, help with his pain and his other symptoms, whether or not he chose to get chemo. They didn't ask about the future, and none of us spoke the D-word; but it was in plain sight between us. Enough said.

We did give Brian chemo, but it didn't slow things down any. We kept him comfy while he lived out his last weeks, and *the three of them each seemed to accept things. Death was never mentioned in front of him that I know of, but Brian seemed to relax and welcome my visits, while his parents pressed me privately with questions about how the end would be, what they could do, and what to tell him. Did you ever get to ask those kinds of questions, Mummy?*

I came to see that no question had an answer I could have learned in medical school. But I kept relearning the big lesson: listen more than talk. And I can only think your death, and the way the communications were handled, played a huge part in shaping me as a doctor.

Your loving son,
John.

How to talk about death and dying is only now getting into medical school curricula, and medical students still get little training in how to break bad news. To do it well asks a capacity for close connection between doctor and patient, which must come not from our technical training but from our hearts—meaning heart in its ancient sense as the place where intellect and emotion, spirit and will, converge. The best doctors are those who bring "compassionate objectivity" to their work. The word servant comes from the Greek *theraps*, from which we get therapist. But servant also means attendant, and nowadays that label gets attached to us—the attending physician. Which is the greatest gift my mother gave me—that of being entirely present for the first twelve years of my life. She utterly rejected the possibility of going out to work for her living, let alone to advance her career, to raise us. She put her whole brilliant self into the art of mothering, in the largest sense, in our formative years. The most holistic form of education and care there can be.

I've spent much of my career trying to bring my whole self to the workplace—body, mind and spirit. Achieving this means bringing my spiritual values to every patient and family encounter. Being a Quaker has taught me belief in "spirit medicine," and I'm no longer shy about declaring my work as God-given. So it's great to see that most medical schools now have coursework not just on death and dying, but on spirituality in medicine. Since I had no such mentors, I've learned pretty much everything I know from my patients—by paying good attention to these young people, listening well, and finding out what works. And thank heaven for humor in hard situations: it can sometimes make the unbearable bearable. Patch Adams says, "Show me the evidence that solemnity ever cured anything!" And to paraphrase G.K. Chesterton, children, like angels, can fly because they take themselves lightly.

I reflect on all the young people who were my early teachers. Seven-year-old Dorothy and her mother in my Finals *viva voce*, who helped me overcome my deep fear of sick children. Jeffrey, the wisecracking stevedore who taught me the power of humor to help us face the horrors of unrelenting illness. Tim, the twelve-year-old with cystic fibrosis, whom I met at the very start of my pediatric training. Audrey, my first child with cancer, who taught me the power of children to respond almost instantaneously to chemo, and to bounce back into life. Ilena, the eighteen-year-old Greek Cypriot, who took such pride in being the first girl with thalassemia to menstruate. Annie, the fourteen-year-old who gave birth to premie twins in Glasgow, whose babies taught me about human resilience when the odds were so heavily stacked against them. And Gena, who taught me the healing power of prayer.

In the heyday of letter-writing in the nineteenth century, letters must have arrived on the doorstep with the expectation of a reply. So perhaps I shouldn't have been surprised to receive a prompt one from Mummy. Three weeks after I'd written her, my sister Elizabeth's husband, Malcolm, died after a long illness. Back at her house after the funeral, Elizabeth produced a letter with a George VI British stamp on the envelope, and the date and place of mailing clearly visible: "Weston-super-Mare, 31/12/54."

"John, I've done a lot of sorting since Malcolm died," Elizabeth tells me, "and I was going through all these boxes that have lain undisturbed for years. I came across this unopened letter dating back to 1954. Isn't it amazing? It even talks about Mummy wanting you to become a doctor."

"My goodness, I don't remember a single conversation in which she brought up that idea. But the really astonishing thing is that I wrote my own letter to her just a few weeks back, telling her all about what I ended up doing with my life."

I open the letter. It reads in part,

> *My darling Elizabeth, Mary, Jane and John, my best beloveds,*
> *I shall not be far away from you, always watching your proud achievements . . . John, I hope you set your goal early on,*

and go for it. I think you will choose Medicine. . . . remember the two principles I instilled in you—Faith and Fortitude.

God Bless you, Mummy.

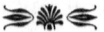

ACKNOWLEDGMENTS

Such a host of people I've come to know in a half-century of medicine—learning, teaching, practicing. I see you in my mind's eye, though many of your names are gone. Most especially, children—you who are no longer with us, and you who have grown to adulthood, often to create families of your own—you are the heroes of this book. I always gave my best for you—though it was little against all you gave me. My grown-up mentors, thank you for your instruction, friendship, trust, especially my countless friends, students, colleagues in London, Norwich, Glasgow, Cleveland, and Gainesville.

Treasured artist friends, my abiding love and gratitude to you. I see all your shining faces—too many to name. Art is as vital to our healing as science, and you have constantly blessed those in your care with your creativity, joy, and wisdom.

I took five years to write this book—with editors coming to my aid at every step. Dorothy, our talks-that-never-ended, from morning kitchen to nighttime bedroom, first sparked me to get this story down, and continued to enrich its content and expression. Ruth and Sheila, you were so much a part of it—thank you for your companionship, your acceptance, even your forgiveness.

Anne Louise MacDonald, Angus MacCaul, John Reeves, Peter Smith—my astute and oh-so-gentle writing group—you never forgot what bits I'd already read you, many times, always spotted another nuance to tweak. Anne Camozzi and Marcia Trahan, your discernment and vision lifted my writing off the page, pinpointing abundant ways to better it. Finally, Heather Tosteson at Wising Up Press, heartfelt thanks for committing to publish Journeys with a Thousand Heroes, and guiding me through those crucial refining steps to market. You knew how to polish my last drafts to make it as good as it could be.

Thank you all for helping me grow closer in understanding to myself. And Florence Doreen—Mummy—my heart is yours always. You gifted me any eloquence to be found here.

DISCUSSION QUESTIONS

CHAPTER 1: LEAVING

1. The formative experience of John Graham-Pole's childhood was the death of his mother from cancer when he was twelve—not only the death itself but also the way people around him responded to it. How was serious illness or death presented to you as a child by the adults around you? Does that experience continue to shape your attitudes about illness and death?

2. Did it surprise you that John decided to go to medical school when he had no intrinsic intellectual curiosity about science? Do you think of the study and practice of medicine as inspired primarily by a scientific bent? What do you think were the major influences on his decision to pursue medicine—family tradition, economic opportunity in the form of a scholarship, observing his uncle at work as a local general practitioner?

3. John's medical education was almost completely subsidized by scholarships. How true do you think that is for American physicians today?

4. Does the motto "See one, do one, teach one" make you feel secure as a patient? What are the benefits to the medical students, as doctors in training, of immediately applying the procedures they learn on real people? What intellectual and emotional skills does this approach encourage? What ones does it discourage?

CHAPTER 2: JOURNEYING

5. Many of the stories in this chapter are told, often humorously, from the point of view of an anxious, sometimes inept, young intern on a steep learning curve. How would these events have looked from the point of view of the person receiving the lumbar puncture or waiting for a successful venipuncture?

6. What were the norms of cancer treatment in the mid-60s in Britain in terms of informed consent? What was John learning during his internship about how to interact with patients? Honesty? Shared responsibility? Right to know?

CHAPTER 3: MAKING FRIENDS
7. Why do you think John finds it easier to interact with children suffering from cancer than adults, including the children's parents?

8. Communication about diagnosis and prognosis are handled far more directly at Jenny Lind Children's Hospital than they were on the adult wards. But is there equal directness about the basis for and consequences of treatment decisions? In the case of Audrey, how honestly do the doctors discuss with her parents the highly experimental nature of the treatment they are suggesting? Children can tolerate more drugs, which makes them more informative from a scientific standpoint when trying new drug therapies, even if their long-term prognosis is no better than for adults. Is this an adequate reason to test unproven therapies on them?

9. What attempts are made to include the child in the decision-making? John says, "None of us have tried to tell Audrey anything about what had struck her down but she seems to have a blind acceptance of how her life is unfolding. Perhaps this is how children deal with things quite beyond their control." Do you think children should or should not be included in such decisions? In what situations and at what ages?

CHAPTER 4: LEARNING
10. Is there a shift in the tone of the memoir as John begins to focus in his specialty? Does it have to do with his attitude toward his work, his mentors, or his patients? What do you think has changed?

CHAPTER 5: CLIMBING
11. John's career takes off after his time in Glasgow. He becomes conversant with cutting edge American technologies, particularly the continuous flow cell separator, which opens up new treatments for leukemia. It also opens up new moral dilemmas. For example, he decides to use a father's white blood cells to help treat his desperately ill son, Will, without informing the father

that the treatment had never been tried before, admitting only after the treatment has been successfully conducted, that "you were what we might call guinea pigs." Do you think you would have reacted as the father in this story if you had been informed in this way, even if the treatment was successful?

12. Nurse K, the head nurse on the ward, questions the use of these new cancer therapies because she does not believe they justify the intense suffering that is involved for the child whereas John emphasizes their curative promise. Later John raises moral questions about physicians on Harley Street treating hopeless cases at great expense. At these points in his career, how would you describe his sense of the kinds of responsibility a physician has to his patients? What are your reactions to these dilemmas and how they were handled?

CHAPTER 6: VENTURING

13. This chapter covers a period of great personal change, much of it dramatic and chaotic, including a marital break-up, and the decision not only to change jobs but also to emigrate to the U.S. Does our evaluation of the professional competency of our physicians change with our evaluation of their private choices? Does it change more than our evaluation of the competence of other professionals, for example lawyers or teachers? Should it?

14. What are the most difficult dimensions for John of adjusting to how Americans practice medicine?

15. In Cleveland, John again becomes interested in promising but very high risk and untried cancer therapies, stem-cell transplants and high-dose chemo treatments. All treatments have risk associated with them, but what makes some people weight their assessments more toward the benefits of intervention and experimentation?

CHAPTER 7: GROUNDING

16. As John and his colleagues try to set up a stem cell transplant unit at the University of Florida's Shands Hospital, they face pushback because of the experimental nature of the treatment, its very high cost, and its potential toxicity. Do you think that at that time, as a doctor, a hospital administrator, or parent of a young patient you would have been supportive or dismissive of their efforts? What concerns would you raise?

17. John describes their need to attract patients to the new unit to keep the beds filled. Is the extent of such business concerns in U.S. hospitals and the practice of medicine a concern to you or do you think of it as an unavoidable practical necessity?

18. This chapter presents us explicitly with a wide range of moral questions about informed consent that face all physicians, but especially pediatricians:

- The decision to have Joseph, a boy with thalassemia who could have lived ten more years without radical treatment, undergo stem cell treatment that is ultimately unsuccessful, the decision explained to parents with rudimentary English through a translator.
- Ed, treated several times for childhood cancer, who now as a young man insists on being an active participant in any treatment decisions—and as a psychology student directly takes on the physicians role in influencing consent.
- Kyle, who at ten knows he wants to stop treatments.
- Brendon and Malila, sixteen year old parents, who decide at their doctor's suggestion to enter their newborn in a clinical trial.
- John's own decision to leave all medical and surgical decisions concerning his own corneal transplant up to his doctor.

Which of these situations spoke to you most? Why? If you disagreed with a decision made, how would you have acted differently as a physician or as a patient?

Chapter 8: Creating

19. In this chapter we see the impact on patients and the entire hospital community of introducing art into the hospital experience. What were some of the examples of this expanding inclusion of art that were most interesting to you? Have you ever been invited to bring art into your own experiences of being a patient or a healthcare provider? What was the impact for you? For those around you?

20. Does introducing art in healing and spirituality in healing feel like a related and natural progression to you? Would you feel safer putting your physical health in the hands of someone who talked to you about these dimensions of your experience of illness or care?

Chapter 9: Homecoming

21. At the end of his career, John's interest turns to end-of-life care, hospice for pediatric patients. Given his aggressive use of radical therapies to preserve life even at great cost, what psychological shifts does this change in focus to dying with grace require? How has he changed from the twelve year old who sat helpless at his mother's death bed vowing to beat cancer?

22. John keeps loyal and tender vigil for thirty-six hours at the bed of a dying sixteen-year-old girl, Ella, at her request. She has decided to refuse further treatment against her grief-stricken parents wishes and wants his support. Does a physician only have primary responsibility to the patient or to the whole family system when we are dealing with the death of a child? Are there other choices of how to handle this situation that could have respected Ella's wishes and also have helped her parents stay close to their daughter during her dying hours?

23. Finishing this memoir of a doctor's career at the cutting edge of a very difficult, risky, often heart-rending specialty, do you feel a greater empathy for doctors? A stronger need for a more holistic approach to medicine? A stronger need to make more informed decisions?

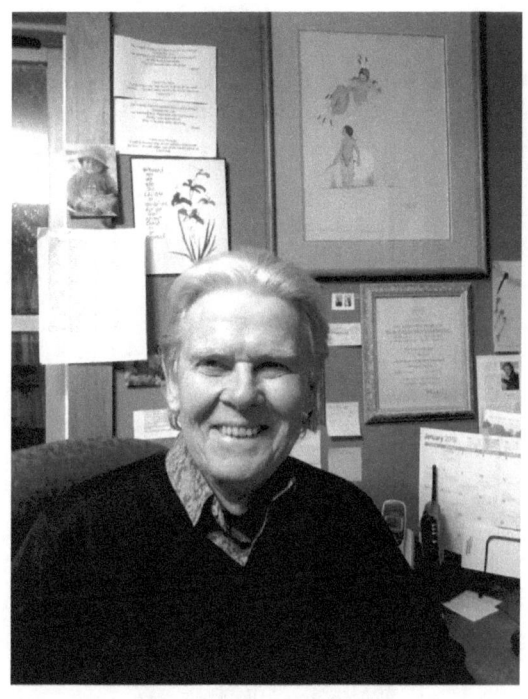

Dr. John Graham-Pole is a retired professor of pediatrics. Originally educated in the United Kingdom, he has been a clinician, teacher and pioneer researcher in the field of childhood cancer for over twenty-five years in the U.S. In 1991, he co-founded Arts in Medicine at the University of Florida, one of the nation's leading university hospital arts program. As well as over 120 scientific publications, he has published poems and essays on the healing arts, and is author of *Illness and the Art of Creative Self-Expression*. He also performs as an improvisational actor and clown. He has been a board member for several national organizations, including the American Holistic Medical Association, Society for Arts in Healthcare and the National Association for Poetry Therapy. He currently lives in Antigonish, Nova Scotia. His website is www.johngrahampole.com, and he can be found on Facebook and Twitter (@GpPole). To order this book: www.universaltable.org/bookstore.html

ILLNESS & MEANING

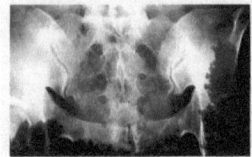

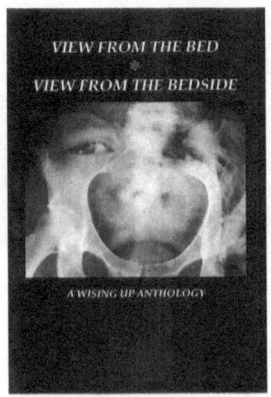

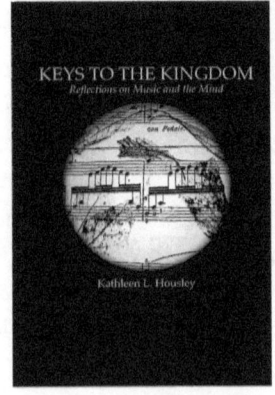

OTHER BOOKS FROM WISING UP PRESS

WISING UP PRESS COLLECTIVE

Only Beautiful & Other Stories
Live Your Life & Other Stories
My Name Is Your Name & Other Stories
Kerry Langan

Keys to the Kingdom: Reflections on Music and the Mind
Epiphanies
Kathleen L. Housley

Last Flight Out: Living, Loving & Leaving
Phyllis A. Langton

A Hymn that Meanders
Maria Nazos

Germs of Truth
Visible Signs
The Philosophical Transactions of Maria van Leeuwenhoek, Antoni's Dochter
Heather Tosteson

WISING UP ANTHOLOGIES

SURPRISED BY JOY
THE KINDNESS OF STRANGERS
SIBLINGS: *Our First Macrocosm*
CREATIVITY & CONSTRAINT
CONNECTED: *What Remains as We All Change?*
DARING TO REPAIR: *What Is It, Who Does It & Why?*
VIEW FROM THE BED, VIEW FROM THE BEDSIDE
LOVE AFTER 70
ILLNESS &GRACE, TERROR & TRANSFORMATION

www.universaltable.org
wisingup@universaltable.org
P.O. Box 2122
Decatur, GA 30031-2122

www.ingramcontent.com/pod-product-compliance
Lightning Source LLC
Chambersburg PA
CBHW030853170426
43193CB00009BA/588